Mentoring Nursing and Healthcare Students

David Kinnell and Phillip Hughes

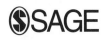

Los Angeles | London | New Delhi
Singapore | Washington DC

SAGE Publications Ltd
1 Oliver's Yard
55 City Road
London EC1Y 1SP

SAGE Publications Inc.
2455 Teller Road
Thousand Oaks, California 91320

SAGE Publications India Pvt Ltd
B 1/I 1 Mohan Cooperative Industrial Area
Mathura Road
New Delhi 110 044

SAGE Publications Asia-Pacific Pte Ltd
33 Pekin Street #02-01
Far East Square
Singapore 048763

Library of Congress Control Number: 2009927728

British Library Cataloguing in Publication data

A catalogue record for this book is available from the British Library.

ISBN 978-1-84787-325-5
ISBN 978-1-84787-326-2 (pbk)

Typeset by C&M Digitals (P) Ltd, Chennai, India
Printed by Biddles, Bodmin, Cornwall
Printed on paper from sustainable resources

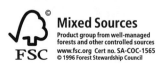

Mixed Sources
Product group from well-managed
forests and other controlled sources
www.fsc.org Cert no. SA-COC-1565
© 1996 Forest Stewardship Council

FSC

Contents

List of boxes, figures and tables

Boxes

Figures

Tables

Introduction

David Kinnell

The format of this book

Mentorship provides a unique opportunity for healthcare personnel to influence the next generation of professionals and ultimately the development of their specific profession. Mentor preparation training programmes, and the subsequent annual mentor updates that are required by the Nursing and Midwifery Council (NMC) (2008a) help mentors to gain an awareness of the role and to maintain currency of their knowledge. Therefore, the fascination of mentorship lies with the challenges that the role entails and the realization that the mentor needs to see mentorship from both perspectives – the mentor and the student.

The rationale for producing this book is to capitalize on experiences gained while supporting mentors who undertake mentor training and subsequently are proactive in maintaining their own mentor update. In August 2006, the NMC introduced their document, *Standards to Support Learning and Assessment in Practice: NMC Standards for Mentors, Practice Teachers and Teachers* with the intention that the content would influence all mentor preparation training programmes as from September 2007. Therefore, this book explores those recommendations and offers an interpretation of their implementation, focusing on the second edition of the standards printed in July 2008.

Despite the focus relating specific to nursing and midwifery, the intention is to adopt a more generic interprofessional throughout by comparing the NMC (2008a) guidelines with those stated by the Health Professions Council (HPC) (2007a; 2007b). The ideology of contemporary healthcare encourages a professional partnership between nursing, midwifery and the supporting allied professions as all those involved in delivering care will contribute to the patient's healthcare journey. The more effective this interrelatedness is and the more coherent the understanding of each health profession's role, the more effective the care given to the patient should be.

The aim of this book therefore is to reflect on that nursing, midwifery and health professions alliance and how each healthcare professional undertakes a vital role throughout the patient's experience of healthcare. In order to assist healthcare students to understand their role while in the practice placement, they will be assigned a mentor, who is a registered nurse, midwife or health professional registrant. All healthcare professions undertaking their role are guided by the recommendations stipulated by the Nursing and Midwifery Council for nurses and midwives or the Health Professions Council for other allied profession registrants. This professional partnership should lead to a safe and successful healthcare experience for the patient throughout their medical journey, irrespective of the specific pathway.

Throughout the book, the term 'healthcare student' will be adopted in order to present a generalized approach applicable to nursing, midwifery and allied health professions. There is a belief that although the guidelines are from the NMC, a more generalized appreciation of the content should be addressed, so the contrast with the HPC will be emphasized where applicable, in order to promote this book as a useful educational resource for all professionals who mentor healthcare students.

Throughout this book the underpinning ideology is to examine the roles and responsibilities of the mentor, and how they enhance the process of mentorship. Each chapter will adopt a generalized approach focused on the chapter title, the discussion will highlight how these general principles and practices of mentorship can be transferable to nursing, midwifery or other health professionals. A number of underpinning theoretical concepts are identified throughout that are based on traditional theories or knowledge generated from significant research studies. Therefore, irrespective of the specialist profession of the healthcare student, the book will offer some generic principles that will provide a starting point to enhance the transition from a registered nurse or midwife to a qualified mentor.

Overview of the chapters

Chapter 1 provides an overview of the mentor's role, its adoption and development in the education of healthcare professionals. It will examine the qualities and skills of an effective mentor and, conversely, discuss the complexities of mentorship. The Nursing and Midwifery Council (2006a) specified the eight domains for mentorship that should be introduced nationally and used from a generalized perspective as from September 2007. The revised domains (NMC, 2008a) will be presented as the linchpin throughout each chapter because of their generic implications.

However, this book is not intended for nurses or midwives alone. It is hoped that while much of the background is from a nursing and midwifery origin, it will also be useful to other health profession registrants. Therefore, reference will be made throughout to the Health Professions Council (2007a). The common denominator for all professions is the need to examine and explore the working relationships in the healthcare setting, based on mutual trust and respect. The focus of Chapter 2 will highlight the importance of group dynamics, and the significance of individual inter-personal variables on the impact of mentorship. The topic of communication and inter-personal skills is usually one of the first topics that the student nurse encounters during their first few weeks of basic nurse training. However, the importance of this subject is also pertinent to midwifery and other health professions. This chapter will offer a brief review of some significant intra-personal concepts including attitudes, emotions, and the self-concept. These may be some of the main topics discussed in pre-registration programmes or part of mentor training because they can also be related to the understanding of the relationship between the mentor and the healthcare student. Mentors may wish to consider these topics if they are trying to understand their student's behaviour – this could be a useful starting point.

One of the most accredited responsibilities of mentors, irrespective of specific profession, is their ability to facilitate learning for healthcare students. Chapter 3 will examine the process of learning and the associated underpinning theoretical concepts. In order to assist mentors to understand the individuality of their student's approach to learning, the concepts of learning styles, learning theories, and what enhances or inhibits learning, will be considered. Throughout this chapter, the discussion will focus on a number of significant concepts that can also offer an explanation of mentorship. It is important for mentors to explore their own practice placement and objectively evaluate its effectiveness in encouraging self-directed learning for adult learners before they consider another integral function of mentorship, the assessment of learning.

In Chapter 4, the process of mentorship will be explored, highlighting that mentors are expected to assess their students using criterion referencing – a set of competencies, outcomes or proficiencies that have been established by an academic governing body. The chapter will discuss the process of assessment using a five-dimensional model that has been designed to assist mentors in the practice placements. The process of assessment should be objective but, unfortunately, for several reasons, there are a number of associated complexities. The reasons why assessments may be problematic will be examined and this will encourage mentors to review their own assessment skills in an attempt to ensure that they are not being subjective. Assessment is a challenge for mentors but nevertheless is certainly one of the most rewarding aspects inherent in the role. This Chapter includes a number of activities, scenarios and frequently asked questions that highlight that mentorship is challenging for both mentor and the healthcare student. From a nursing perspective, the mentor has always been accountable to the NMC for their judgement regarding a student's achievement, and this commitment continues.

The importance of Chapter 5 is that it ascertains the effectiveness of facilitation of learning and the process of assessment. As these are two major components of mentorship, it is educationally viable to gain feedback to ensure what is being delivered is meeting the healthcare students' needs. Throughout this chapter, issues such as students' evaluation of placement, clinical audits and discussions between students and mentors will be explored. The overarching theme is directed towards ensuring the practice placement is an appropriate environment conducive to student learning.

As a continuity strategy, what makes an 'effective' placement for healthcare students will be the exploratory theme throughout Chapter 6. The practice placement is a vital setting for ensuring that the healthcare student can relate theory to practice. It is therefore essential that mentors review the effectiveness of their placements and evaluate the provision of academic learning resources that are available for students to access. This will depend on the speciality and type of student accessing the healthcare setting but a positive commitment is advantageous if the process of mentorship is going to be student-centred. The theme context of practice attempts to identify specific individuality characteristics that make the student the person that they are.

Chapter 7 relates to the previous one and emphasizes the importance of ensuring that care delivery is appropriate to meeting contemporary healthcare. The outcomes focus on the importance of interprofessional partnership and ensuring the environment reflects that contemporary ideology to enhancing learning. Therefore, the focus throughout will examine issues such as welcoming students into the practice placement, the importance of the tripartite interviews, helping them to achieve the 'essential skills clusters' assessments and to identify the importance of disability equality training for mentors. Some of these contemporary changes are in response to increasing awareness of evidence-based practice.

For all nurses, midwives and health professions there is a need to ensure that their own personal and professional knowledge, skills and attitudes represent a pro-active contemporary stance. Throughout Chapter 8, the focus is directed towards lifelong learning and ensuring that the importance of research-based practice is acknowledged and implemented wherever appropriate. Therefore, an overview of research methodologies, and differentiation between quantitative and qualitative research approaches will emphasise nurses' awareness of evidence-based practice within contemporary healthcare and particularly mentorship.

The aim throughout Chapter 9 is to review the process of mentorship and those involved in providing a support network. This includes a review of leadership skills, how these link to the new approach to mentorship and the impact of managing change in the contemporary NHS. The updated ten-day mentor training programme and the need for annual mentor updates will be explored in order to meet the NMC (2008a) recommendations. An overview of the triennial reviews and the future introduction of the sign-off mentor will also be explored and the additional responsibilities highlighted.

The final chapter is unique because it offers a summary of the reality of mentorship and how mentors have actually dealt with the differences between idealism and reality in respect of their role. The importance of phenomenology for generating new research-based data will be explored. Throughout, it is hoped that new mentors undertaking a mentor preparation training programme will be able to focus on their own development of 'becoming a mentor' and how the eight domains, and 26 outcomes have been used as a supportive guiding framework.

How to use this book

This book is a valuable guide for those nurses who, following registration, will be working towards gaining an insight into mentorship at Stage One: Nurses and Midwives level and then continuing to undertake mentor preparation training in order to become a Stage Two: Mentor. In each chapter, the NMC (2008a) aims and outcomes for both stages will be identified and form the basis for the remainder of the chapter. The overall content will help mentors to relate the identified underpinning theoretical perspectives to the process of mentorship so that they can apply the content to their own practice placement.

Also, the book will be helpful for all existing mentors in order to encourage them to be introspective, explore their own mentorship experiences and be utilised as an educational tool to enhance their annual mentor update. Throughout 2008, the NMC introduced or revised a number of changes to mentorship and other aspects of the nursing profession, and a number of these will be explored throughout the book. Each chapter contains a number of thought-provoking features: Mentor Activities, case studies and frequently asked questions that are intended to generate discussion between all mentors. By engaging in these discussions, this will result in a sharing of ideas and experiences so that those at the Stage One: Nurses and Midwives level can value the Stage Two: Mentor's lived experience of mentorship.

The Mentor Activities are designed both for self-reflection or to be discussed with colleagues, depending on the construction of your work team. The case studies are genuine and are a combination of both positive and negative mentorship experiences which will assist mentors to gain an awareness of the challenges and sense of achievement that mentorship entails. Each case study will end with a thought-provoking question to reflect on individually or discuss with your colleagues. This book will have its most vital role as a complementary or essential text to support the five educational input days associated with mentor preparation training, depending on the stance taking. Each chapter will focus on one of the eight domains specified by the NMC (2008a) so that if the student cannot attend a school-based day for whatever reason, the corresponding chapter can be used as a self-directed mechanism that will meet the learning outcomes for that day. The presentational syntax throughout the book is in the format of an ongoing discussion similar to that undertaken in the classroom. This was the format suggested by those undertaking mentor training and as part of mentor update discussions when the proposal for writing this book was suggested. This approach of relating theory to practice was identified as being user friendly for 'busy' mentors.

Therefore, this book will be a valuable educational resource and pertinent to a wide audience of healthcare professionals because:

1   It adopts an interprofessional approach, focusing on advisory guidelines from the Nursing and Midwifery Council, as well as the Health Professions Council.
2   It encourages an exploration of both the mentor's role as well as that of the healthcare student. This approach will encourage an awareness and appreciation of each other's subsequent role while contributing to the delivery of care to patients at the various stages of their healthcare journey.
3   This is a valuable text for all those undertaking mentor training or wishing to update their own knowledge of contemporary mentorship in accordance with the requirements stated by the NMC (2008a).
4   It will hopefully be used as a useful discussion educational resource for existing mentors, particularly if you engage in all the Mentor Activities, case studies and frequently asked questions.

1

Mentoring nursing and healthcare students

David Kinnell

Introduction

In contemporary healthcare, there is a need to appreciate the importance of the interprofessional partnership that exists between nurses, midwives and other health professions. In higher education institutes, healthcare students from nursing, midwifery and other allied professions are encouraged to explore the patient's healthcare journey and all those involved in its various stages. A number of different healthcare personnel may be involved throughout that patient's healthcare journey, nevertheless, it is important to appreciate the roles and responsibilities of all those involved. Throughout this chapter an overview of the development and implementation of the mentor's roles and responsibilities will be explored and how they can assist healthcare students appreciate the patient's experience by sharing and imparting the knowledge, skills and professional attitudes that they have developed during their own professional career.

The development of mentorship

In the *NHS Next Stage Review* (NSR) for England (DH, June 2008) Lord Darzi stated that quality is the organizing principle for all health services and summarized the challenges being faced as:

- rising patient expectations;
- demographic changes leading to new demands on healthcare system;

- the continuing development of the 'information society';
- advances in treatments;
- the changing nature of disease;
- changing expectations of the health workplace. (NHS Connecting for Health, 2009: 6)

This summarizes a contemporary approach to healthcare delivery that all nurses, midwives and allied professions have to acknowledge in order to improve the 'quality' of experience that patients are exposed to. So not only have healthcare professionals a duty to respond to changes in the National Health Service, they should also have a commitment to nurse education. Mentorship is the process that allows the transference of knowledge, skills and attitudes from health professionals to the students that they are working with.

It may be interesting for some mentors to understand how the role has evolved and the various definitions and connotations that have attributed to what has become a vital, supportive and educational role. Mentoring has for the past 15 years been high on the agenda for the consistency in the preparation and support of healthcare students. Allan et al. (2008) trace the historical development of the mentorship role and how the relationship has evolved in response to how the students' role in the practice setting has changed since the 1970s. Indeed, students were then the main care givers and by doing so, learnt from hands-on experience.

> Moores and Moult (1979) estimated 75% of direct care used to be given by students in the 1970's and trained nurses taught and students learned while they worked (Fretwell, 1982); at least until the curriculum reforms of the 1980's and the introduction of supernumerary practice for students with the Project 2000 curriculum. (Allan et al., 2008: 546)

The introduction of the Project 2000 programme in the early 1990s emphasized how important the mentor was within nurse education and for ensuring the importance of relating theory to practice. The role and importance of the mentor within practice placements have continued to develop and become highly respected by healthcare students. The mentor guides the student and hopefully shares with them their knowledge and skills that they have acquired so the student can benefit from their experiences.

The aim of this professional relationship is to facilitate and enhance the student's learning, as the more able they are, the more effective the transition from student to professional will be, ensuring their fitness for practice at the point of registration (Moore, 2005). This also acknowledges their new career which will hopefully allow them to be able to support and prepare other healthcare students on their journey to qualification.

This applies to all nursing, midwifery and allied professions, therefore the generic term 'healthcare student' will be used throughout in order to reflect the interprofessional approach to learning that is encouraged in practice placements in today's healthcare provision service.

Although the aim of this book is to adopt a contemporary concept, the idea of mentorship has its origins in Greek literature (see Box 1.1).

Box 1.1   Historical account of the origins of mentorship

In Greek literature it is written in Homer's *Odyssey,* according to Morton-Cooper and Palmer (2000), that 'Mentor', the son of Alimus, was assigned by Ulysses to be a tutor-adviser to look after his son Telemachus, whilst he was away fighting the Trojan wars on behalf of his kingdom.

Ulysses was away far longer than anticipated so Mentor had a great deal of influence on Telemachus' education and upbringing.

The correlation is that the important and valued role of contemporary mentors ensures that they also help to educate and guide the student throughout their practice placement experiences.

This brief summary shows that mentorship is not a new phenomenon. Mentor came to mean and be synonymous with 'wise and trusted one'. So important was this that in ancient history, the Roman army adopted mentors to develop their soldiers. Mentorship and mentoring seemed to experience a revival in the 1980s in American literature and later in the UK, being associated with business, education and nursing. Also related is the association of adult developmental psychology and its influence within healthcare delivery wherever there is a holistic approach to care and understanding of the person. Within healthcare the patients' physical status is important, particularly when there is an altered health state when this is often the reason why they are receiving care services. However, in contemporary healthcare a more concerted effort is also made to value who the person is (their psychology) and their social background (sociology). Mentors are often involved in helping the student to establish how theoretical concepts help to understand the reality of the interrelatedness of these three aspects of individuality (NMC, 2008b).

The term 'mentor' was connected with adult developmental psychology and the controversial yet well-known research undertaken by Levinson, Darrow, Klein, Levinson and McKee in 1978. Levinson et al. focused their research on *The Seasons of a Man's Life,* highlighting the importance of different time spans in an adult man's development. Their main contribution to the knowledge base was the concept of time spans or eras that represented a period of stable development (referred to as structure building) and transitional phases (or structure changing) (Gross, 2005).

The advantage of Levinson et al.'s (1978) contribution was the notion of a holistic appreciation of the person. The predominant influence was the interaction between biological influences and social experiences resulting in the psychological status of the person. However, the experiences developed from family and work contributions are paramount to life structure and the growth of individuality. Adult developmental psychology is influenced by experiences gained at different phases lasting approximately five years. Levinson et al. contribute to mentorship because, according to their theory, a mentor was someone older and wiser who capitalized on their structure building experiences and offered valued contributions to a younger person. This is a concept that has value to healthcare, for nursing, midwifery and the allied professions.

In 1999, the United Kingdom Central Council for Nursing, Midwifery and Health Visiting (UKCC) responded to criticisms regarding the Diploma in Nursing Programme which indicated that students on registration were 'too academic' and not 'very practical'. So, in response to this criticism, the UKCC commissioned Sir Leonard Peach to undertake an independent investigation in order to identify to what extent the concerns were justified. The resultant document *Fitness for Practice* (UKCC, 1999) was not as critical as anticipated. One of the recommendations of the Peach Report was that 'universities and care providers should collaborate to offer nursing students seamless learning opportunities based on the UKCC's existing principles of competence and knowledge acquisition' (Sines et al., 2006: 28).

Contrary to anticipated negative responses, there were a number of determinants that actually enhanced the effectiveness of students achieving fitness for practice at the point of registration (see Box 1.2). Throughout their basic nurse training, mentors are collectively a valued influence in ensuring that the healthcare student is achieving what is expected of them, in correlation with the specific training programme and level of training. The determinants identified are an added perspective.

Box 1.2   Key determinants for achieving fitness for practice at the point of registration

- Implementation of a host trust concept, whereby nursing students are sponsored by dedicated trusts for most of their education programmes.
- Confirmation of learning outcomes at the end of the common foundation programme and determination of standards of proficiency for entry to the register at the end of the branch programme.

- The duration of the common foundation programme was subsequently reduced from 18 to 12 months.
- The development of new partnership models of practice, including multi-professional learning opportunities. (Sines et al., 2006)

Mentors now have to be aware of the NHS Institute for Innovation and Improvement (2006) *NHS Leadership Qualities Framework*. This NHS framework identifies fifteen qualities that range from personal, cognitive, and social quality attributes. These attributes are further segmented into three clusters: personal qualities, setting direction and delivering the service. From the mentor's perspective this framework helps the professional to reflect on their own mentorship skills and to evaluate how they are effectively meeting the qualities highlighted by the NHS Institute. Included within the specific 'personal qualities' variables is 'personal integrity' which identifies the need for mentors to act as a role model and have the motivation to continue with developing the service in response to contemporary healthcare needs.

Subsequently a variety of research studies have been undertaken to examine the benefits of the mentor's role. Irrespective of the research approach undertaken, results generally reveal that there is no doubt that the mentor plays an important role in the student's placement experience. Myall et al. (2008) explored the reality of contemporary mentorship and to what extent the initial ideological concepts made an impact in practice. Although the research involved a number of different strategies, the results emphasized the importance of mentorship within contemporary healthcare (see Box 1.3).

Box 1.3   Summary of some of the benefits associated with mentorship

- Mentors assist in the development of quality student placement experiences.
- Mentor is a source of support and helped students feel connected to the placement area.
- Students were welcomed to the practice environment, and treated as valid and legitimate learner.
- Mentors help create opportunities to maximize students' learning.
- Mentors help students to develop their practical skills.
- Mentors felt mentorship provided the opportunity to provide clinical support to students and subsequently helped them to keep their own clinical skills up to date.
- Mentoring helps mentors to achieve a great sense of job satisfaction.
- Mentors felt 'proud' as they watched the student develop their knowledge, skills and professional attitudes. (Myall et al., 2008)

In the list of prerequisites for the role of mentor, the NMC (2008a) state that a qualified nurse should have at least 12 months full-time post-registration experience (or equivalent part-time). This appears to be a realistic and practical requirement. It is during this time that the newly qualified nurse will settle into and get to know their new professional role. Indeed, it is at this time that continued support is needed in the form of preceptorship (Morton-Cooper and Palmer, 2000).

'The Nursing and Midwifery Council is the regulator for two professions: nursing and midwifery. The primary purpose of the NMC is to safeguard the health and wellbeing of the public' (NMC, 2008a: 05). Therefore, whenever the NMC sets standards or issues new guidelines, they are using the procedure to involve nurses and midwives already recorded on the register, in order to gain feedback. These standards are usually in place for five years and reviewed as required. Mentor standards have been subject to such a review and changes have been implemented.

The standards for mentors and mentorship have recently been revised (NMC, 2006a). The revision began in 2003 with a national consultation. Although there had been a delay in the production of the revised standards, they were finally available in August 2006. While it was suggested that these could be implemented as early as September 2006, in some cases this was too brief a time period. The deadline for the revised standards called 'domains' to be implemented across the country was September 2007. This document presents considerably more detail than its predecessor and is now in its second edition, as of July 2008.

Some standards were retained in the new domains whilst others were modified in order to enhance clarity to help the mentor understand their role more effectively. Some generated discussion and appeared to be confusing or even ambiguous. These mentorship standards (NMC, 2008a) are now based on eight domains, have identified specific outcomes and throughout this book each chapter will examine and explore each one (see Table 1.1).

The value in contrasting these two changes is so that mentors who were trained using the NMC (2004a) 'standards' can now compare the differences between those and the latest NMC (2008a) 'domains', appreciating that there is a close similarity. When the new domains were introduced, existing mentors were concerned that there was a vast difference between the two; throughout each chapter the content will reassure mentors that the existing knowledge they have remains valuable and pertinent to contemporary mentorship.

The NMC (2008a) now supports a developmental framework that should be used to map a person's personal and professional development during their post-registration lifelong learning. There are potentially four

TABLE 1.1   *Comparison of the 2004 Standards and the 2008 Domains*

2004 Mentor Standards	2008 Mentor Domains
1 Communication and effective working relationships	1 Establishing effective working relationships
2 Facilitation of learning	2 Facilitation of learning
3 Assessment	3 Assessment and accountability
4 Role modelling	4 Evaluation of learning
5 Creating an environment for learning	5 Creating an environment for learning
6 Improving practice	6 Context of practice
7 A knowledge base	7 Evidence-based practice
8 Course development	8 Leadership

Note: Within the 2008 domains there are 14 outcomes for the Stage 1: Nurses and Midwives and 26 outcomes for the Stage 2: Mentor.

stages involved in developing the knowledge, skills and attitudes that are required to mentor healthcare students (see Box 1.4).

Box 1.4   The developmental framework for mentors

Stage One: All nurses and midwives following registration.
Stage Two: Standards for mentors following appropriate mentor training.
Stage Three: Standard for a practice teacher for nursing or specialist community public health nursing.
Stage Four: Standards for a teacher of nurses, midwives or specialist community public health nursing.

Stage One: Nurses and Midwives

Stage One is an introduction to the roles and responsibilities of being a mentor. The underpinning philosophy relates to the previous NMC (2004b), clause 6.4 which states: 'You have a duty to facilitate students of nursing and midwifery and others to develop their competence.' The same theme has been transferred to the NMC (2008b) *The Code: Standards of Conduct, Performance and Ethics for Nurses and Midwives* which now states that:

You must establish that anyone you delegate to is able to carry out your instructions.

You must make sure that everyone you are responsible for is supervised and supported (p. 6).

You must facilitate students and others to develop their competence (p. 5).

Therefore, once qualified, the nurse or midwife has to work towards completing the eight domains and their associated 14 outcomes related to Stage One. During this time, they have completed their preceptorship programme and the requirements for their Knowledge and Skills Framework Portfolio (Department of Health, 2004). The outcomes help mentors from their transition following newly qualified to undertaking a recognized mentor training programme in preparation for becoming a Stage Two mentor.

Stage Two: Mentor

According to the NMC (2008a: 16) 'Nurses and midwives can become a mentor when they have successfully achieved all of the outcomes of this stage.'

There are eight domains and 26 outcomes for Stage Two. There has been a well-established move towards standardizing the basic Mentor Preparation Programme in response to the initial NMC (2006a), and later in 2008, requirements that state there must be a minimum of ten days within which at least five must be protected time to allow for learning, consolidation, and internalizing that knowledge. All Mentor Training Programmes are being validated and given approval by the NMC, but will be revisited in five years time.

The following is an example of how a programme could be implemented but the final arrangements will be set by the specific higher education institute. In response to the NMC (2008a) guidelines, a programme of ten days duration could be organized – one day a week over a ten-week period. On alternate weeks (weeks one, three, five, seven, nine), Stage One mentors attend for direct face-to-face meeting with a lecturer in the School of Nursing to examine the underpinning theoretical concepts associated with the roles and responsibilities of the mentor, based on the eight domains. This involves feedback from work-based learning activities, classroom discussions, group activities and scenario exercises.

The work-based learning activities could be designed to help achieve the identified 26 outcomes and could be completed whilst in the practice setting (weeks two, four, six, eight and ten). Each Stage One mentor is encouraged to work with a colleague (already a Stage Two mentor) who adopts the role of a supporting practice mentor, thereby providing a medium for academic and professional discussions regarding mentoring a student, so that they have 'the opportunity to critically reflect on such an experience' (ibid.: 29). Although ten days is recommended, the NMC state that five of these must be protected time. Throughout this book there are a number of case studies and mentor activities that could be used to enhance this programme and generate mentor discussion.

The NMC (2004c: 34) states that pre-registration students have to develop a student portfolio that provides a range of evidence, to verify their achievements and personal and professional developments whilst in the practice placement. The actual construction of this and what constitutes 'evidence' will be determined by the Higher Education Institute. In order to provide a range of evidence, students can be encouraged, for example, to engage in reflective discussions, reflective writings and collect written support of observed learning whilst attending an insight visit. Therefore, whilst a student nurse is observing a dietitian, occupational therapist, operating department practitioner, physiotherapist, or speech and language therapist, they can complete a statement that reflects their understanding of that health profession's role within the patient's healthcare journey.

The Mentor Preparation Training Programme is usually completed in three months and is usually the only mechanism available for qualified staff undertaking mentor preparation in order to be registered as a Stage Two mentor. It is hoped that mentors now and in the future will feel that they are more effectively prepared for their role, unlike those identified by Andrews and Chilton (2000). However, some nurses may not be mentors by choice but rather undertake the role as a compulsory requirement for their own professional development in order to meet the requirements of the Second Gateway, within the NHS Knowledge and Skills Framework (Royal College of Nursing, 2007a).

There is a marked variation in the way that community, hospital, and independent sector placement staff assist student nurses to feel part of their healthcare team. A Stage One mentor should observe the process of mentorship and the maintenance of an effective learning environment then discuss their observations with a Stage Two mentor in order to help them understand its significance. Student nurses can discuss their experiences on the various placements and then accredit positive feedback to enhance the reputation of that practice placement or identify areas that could be improved. The Stage Two mentor should be viewed as a 'change agent' so must value any feedback in a constructive manner.

Stage Three: Practice Teacher

Stage Three relates to the standards for practice teachers for nursing or specialist public health nursing. Again, there are eight domains, and 26 outcomes, albeit the outcomes are different. An NMC Practice Teacher is a

Registrant who has undertaken a recognized approved Mentor Preparation Programme (equivalent to Stage Two) and then 'received further preparation to achieve the knowledge, skills and competence required to meet the NMC defined outcomes for a practice teacher' (NMC, 2008a: 22).

This is Stage Three in the developmental framework and as a Practice Teacher they are responsible and accountable for:

- organizing and co-ordinating learning activities, primarily in practice learning environments for pre-registration students, and those intending to register as a specialist community public health nurse (SCPHN) and specialist practice qualification, where this is a local requirement;
- supervising students and providing them with constructive feedback on their achievements;
- setting and monitoring achievement of realistic learning objectives in practice;
- assessing total performance – including skills, attitudes and behaviours;
- providing evidence as required by programme providers of the student's achievement or lack of achievement;
- liaising with others (e.g. mentors, sign-off mentors, supervisors, personal tutors, the programme leader, other professionals) to provide feedback and identify any concerns about the student's performance and agree action as appropriate;
- signing off achievement of proficiency at the end of the final period of practice learning or a period of supervised practice (ibid.: 22).

Stage Four: Teacher

In contrast, this stage has specific criteria to achieve and that relates to the standard for a teacher of nurses and midwives. There are eight domains that have 40 outcomes entwined throughout. This Stage Four standard is mandatory for nurses and midwives based and working in higher education institutes and involved in supporting and assessing in practice settings all students undertaking an NMC-approved programme.

According to the NMC (2008a: 25), an NMC teacher is responsible for:

- organizing and co-ordinating learning activities in both academic and practice environments;
- supervising students in learning situations and providing them with constructive feedback on their achievements;
- setting and monitoring achievement of realistic learning objectives in theory and practice;
- assessing performance and providing evidence as required of student achievement.

The NMC (2008a) developmental framework has been designed to provide a career pathway, from the newly qualified nurses and midwives to the more experienced registered mentor who wishes to undertake teacher training in order to have a teaching qualification recorded on the register with the Nursing and Midwifery Council.

However, the overall focus of this book will be intentionally directed towards the Stage One: nurses and midwives and the Stage Two: mentor. It is intended that each chapter will explore the process of mentorship from a generalized perspective, but with a specific focus on one of the NMC (2008a) domains which will be advantageous to all nurses, midwives and allied healthcare professionals. It is envisaged therefore that a general approach will encourage an interprofessional awareness and appreciation of each health professional's role, although the predominant appearance relates to nursing and midwifery.

Fulton et al. (2008) examined an international perspective of mentorship involving the United Kingdom, Norway, Sweden, Portugal, Iceland and Poland when undertaking a project funded by the European Union as a Leonardo de Vinci pilot.

The aim of the project was to produce a framework for a standardized European Mentor Training Programme. They highlighted that there are four main tasks associated with the mentor's role:

* to encourage students to learn *from* practice and to learn *in* practice;
* to assist the student to acquire focused and specific clinical skills;
* to facilitate the professional socialization of nursing students, and
* to assess and evaluate the student's progress whilst working in the practice placement.

It is expected that the student can correlate what has been taught in the School of Nursing with what is witnessed whilst caring for patients, residents or service users in practice. Unfortunately, this has become an unrealistic expectation and one that emphasizes the dichotomy between idealism and reality. Throughout the history of nurse education and its numerous transformations initiated to meet the ever changing practice placements needs, there still remains the criticism that emphasizes the existence of a theory–practice gap. This is a topic usually explored during the Mentor Preparation Programme and an issue examined by numerous authors including Martin and Mitchell (2001); Higginson (2004); and Borlase and Abelson-Mitchell (2008).

However, despite the criticisms, the practice placement still remains the best method of developing nursing knowledge, skills and professional attitudes (Levett-Jones and Lathlean, 2008). This is an expectation that is pertinent to all nursing, midwifery and healthcare students. Therefore, the mentor's role is to assist practice-based development in order that the experience gained may be reflected upon and documented in the student's written assignments. However, because of the subjectivity associated with the process of assessment, it undoubtedly is not without its inherent complexities. It could be argued that a reliable assessment is one that is consistent. That is, two independent assessors deducing the same conclusions about a student's abilities would constitute a reliable assessment. The mentor needs to know what to look for in the learner such as the practical, intellectual, interpersonal and intrapersonal skills.

The process of mentorship is based on a personal relationship between the mentor and the student. Some mentors demonstrate a strong commitment to ensuring their student achieves their potential whilst working in that particular placement. Others adhere to their principles of self-directed learning and appear to offer very little guidance. Irrespective of the style of mentorship, within the eight domains the mentor is relied upon to identify if the student is safe to practise in order to protect the public. This is also advocated by the NMC (2006b) in their *Standards for Preparation and Practice of Supervisors of Midwives.*

The literature clearly identifies that the statutory supervision of midwives has been the normal process for the over a century. According to the NMC (2006b: 3):

> As a modern regulatory practice, statutory supervision of midwives supports protection of the public by:
>
> • promoting best practice and excellence in care
> • preventing poor practice and
> • intervening in unacceptable practice.
>
> Statutory supervision of midwives is a valuable resource for midwives, their employers and the profession because it enables midwives to provide safe and effective care.

Similar to nursing and other allied health professions, the mentor of student midwives has an important role. In addition, because midwives also work with a supervisor who has completed appropriate training to meet the standards for practice of supervisors, the concept of mentorship is an integral component of the midwives' role. In some higher education institutes, pre-registration diploma/degree in nursing students may have the opportunity to gain a short insight practice placement within the midwifery speciality. So the concepts conceptualized within mentorship will hopefully be applicable.

The Health Professions Council

Whereas the NMC is the governing body for nurses and midwives, the Health Professions Council governs the allied professions. The Health

Professions Council is a health regulator who has a responsibility to protect the health and well-being of people who use the services registered with the Council. Its primary function is to protect the public by establishing standards that health professionals have to adhere to. The overall focus relates to health professionals' education, training, behaviour, skills and health. In contrast to newly qualified nurses Stage One role, qualified health professions are identified by the term Registrant.

Currently 13 health professions are regulated by the HPC (2007a) (see Box 1.5).

Box 1.5   Health professions regulated by the HPC

Arts Therapists
Biomedical Scientists
Chiropodists/Podiatrists
Clinical Scientists
Dietitians
Occupational Therapists
Operating Department Practitioners
Orthoptists
Paramedics
Physiotherapists
Prosthesis/Orthotists
Radiographers
Speech and Language Therapists

Each profession regulated by the Health Professions Council has its own specific 'standards of proficiency' and at times the aim is to compare nurses and midwives with the following: dietitians (HPC, 2007c), occupational therapists (HPC, 2007d), operating department practitioners (HPC, 2004), physiotherapists (HPC, 2007e), and speech and language therapists (HPC, 2007f). It is anticipated that this will encourage a generalized awareness of healthcare student's needs, irrespective of their specific health profession. However, the individual allied professional does work in a number of practice placements including local councils, NHS trusts, prisons, private practice and in schools. Wherever the work-based setting for the health professional, the HPC (2007a) does manage their 'fitness for practice'. This is maintained by encouraging all health professions to abide by the *Standards of Conduct, Performance and Ethics* (HPC, 2007b) that contain 16 standards:

- four relate to standards of conduct;
- eight are associated with standards of performance;
- four relate to high standards of ethics.

In March 2009, the Department of Health (DH) announced their intention to implement 'improvements to the regulation of healthcare professionals'. The government hopes that these new measures will improve the regulation and governance of healthcare professionals in order to provide greater reassurance for the public and professionals. The two new reports *Tackling Concerns Nationally* (2009a) and *Tackling Concerns Locally* (2009b) are part of the government reforms of professional regulation in an attempt to raise professional standards and ensure patient safety.

Tackling Concerns Nationally aims to make recommendations on professional regulation and subsequently assure patient safety at a national level. It has been designed to set out regulations for the establishment of the Office of the Health Professions Adjudicator (OHPA) which will examine cases identified that require assessing for fitness to practise for healthcare professionals. The role of the OHPA's Board Members includes the following:

- ensure that the public interest is served at all times;
- ensure that the principles of equality, diversity, fairness and human rights are upheld.

In contrast, *Tackling Concerns Locally* sets out recommendations and principles of best practice to strengthen local NHS arrangements for identifying poor performance among healthcare workers and taking effective action. These two reports must be viewed as a positive step forward to enhancing quality of care delivery which all nursing, midwifery and allied professionals mentors need to acknowledge and share with their students.

For each of the 13 health professions there are specific guidelines on the standards of proficiency that include both generic and specific recommendations. An awareness of these is paramount when mentoring healthcare students from the specific profession. Thus, throughout the book the intention is to explore both general and then specific aspects, so that mentors will have a beneficial academic tool to accentuate their knowledge, understanding and management of the mentorship process.

This is an interesting time for all mentors as they balance changes in their role both nationally and locally. The skills and energy that are needed to carry out the effective role of a mentor should not be taken for granted. All students undertaking NMC-approved pre-registration midwifery training can only be mentored throughout all their training by a sign-off mentor who has completed the appropriate extra training and met the subsequent criteria. The sign-off mentor status will also be required by all mentors working with student nurses in their final practice placement of their pre-registration training programme although the process does not start until April 2010, unless the student is undertaking a shortened training programme (this is discussed in Chapter 9). Now read and reflect on Case study 1.1.

CASE STUDY 1.1

A student nurse returned from their practice placement stating that they were surprised at how successful the process of mentorship works, its value and support that it offers.

The student had met their mentor when they attended a teaching session with some other mentors, as part of their preparation for practice. The mentor had given the group an overview of the nursing speciality and what they expected from the student. This discussion was valuable because the mentors allowed the students the opportunity to ask questions in an attempt to allay their fears about the practice placement.

The most important aspect from this student's feedback was that the mentor did really try to follow what they said they would.

At the start of the placement, the orientation to the placement was successful and followed by the 'initial interview'. This had given the student the opportunity to share with the mentor their action plan, hopes and aspirations of what they wanted to achieve. The mentor was supportive and made every effort to ensure that the student's experience was as effective as possible.

How far does this correspond to your approach to mentorship?

Case study 1.1 is a very successful account of how mentorship can work and help to reassure the student that the mentor is a valuable aid in their practice placement experience. There are many reasons why mentorship is so successful and is often reflected in the positive approach that the individual has to undertaking appropriate training and maintaining their continued commitment.

Watson (2004) reported the results of a study into why qualified nurses attended a mentor training programme and identified the four main reasons as:

- patient-based reasons for doing the course;
- course-based reasons for doing the course;
- doing the course through need rather than choice;
- doing the course for reasons of personal motivation.

Inevitably, there were a number of qualified nurses undertaking mentor training and using the associated qualification as a vehicle for obtaining professional credibility. Nevertheless, no matter the reasons identified, in reality, some mentors do undertake the role and find the student somewhat challenging.

However, there is no doubt that for some mentors the student offers them a challenge and at the same time, represents hard work in the process as they try to balance and juggle the ever increasing roles and responsibilities enforced upon them (Dolan, 2003). This has been an area of interest and concern, and subsequently has formed the basis of a number of research studies. However, Darling (1985) warned of the dangers of mentors becoming 'toxic mentors', i.e. those who fail to develop an effective supportive rapport with the student because they themselves are tired and exhausted, possibly suffering from burnout (Webb and Shakespeare, 2008).

Research has been undertaken from various perspectives:

• What do students want from their mentor?
• What do students want from the practice placement?
• What do mentors want from their students?

Box 1.6 presents some examples of a few significant studies that highlight how important the process of mentorship is and the need to ensure its effectiveness from a nursing, midwifery and interprofessional learning perspective.

Box 1.6   Examples of significant research studies

'Student and mentor perceptions of mentoring effectiveness' (Andrews and Chilton, 2000).

'The support that mentors receive in the clinical setting' (Watson, 2000).

'Assessing practice of student nurses: methods, preparation of assessors and student views' (Calman et al., 2002).

'Assessing student nurse clinical competency: will we ever get it right?' (Dolan, 2003).

'Belongingness: a prerequisite for nursing students' clinical learning' (Levett-Jones and Lathlean, 2008).

The importance of interprofessional learning has been emphasized over the past decade and after some initial resistance, the partnerships are well established in some healthcare settings. Edwards (2001: 1) emphasized that, 'Each doctor, nurse, midwife, allied professional and support staff must understand their own responsibilities and accountability to deliver the best care, and not to harm patients by their actions.' The aim throughout this book is to develop this approach and emphasize where possible how the interrelatedness of healthcare learning can be enhanced for all healthcare students so that they can appreciate this need for 'best care'.

As part of an annual mentor update (2003–8), the following exercise was given in order to gain some feedback and ensure a clear understanding of what support some mentors may need. Throughout this book there will be a number of thought-provoking exercises relating to the reality of mentorship, try Mentor Activity 1.1.

MENTOR ACTIVITY 1.1

As a mentor, what do you expect from the student nurse?

Reflect on this question and make some notes whilst relating to the specific nursing students that you work with.

Mentorship is an important integral role for all healthcare professions. The opportunities that the professional academic role generates are complementary to those gained from undertaking patient care delivery and management. However, it is useful to gain clarity of thought and completing the Mentor Activity 1.1 exercise will help you gain your own self-awareness of your expectations of the healthcare student (see Table 1.2). Compare these responses in Table 1.2 from a number of qualified Stage Two mentors, with your own.

There is no doubt that nurses, midwives and the allied professions have different expectations of what they want from the mentor's role. Bray and Nettleton (2007) report on the findings of a multi-professional research study that involved nurses, midwives and medics, and they identified, the most important roles that an effective mentor undertakes. Mentors and mentees were asked in a questionnaire to identify the most significant attributes that a mentor possesses, from a pre-selected menu of 20 attributes (see Table 1.3).

The results are interesting and, furthermore, thought-provoking. Although there are similarities, it is nevertheless the important role of being a 'teacher' that appears to be most significant. However, the term 'facilitator' may be

TABLE 1.2   *"As a mentor, what do you expect from a student nurse?"*

Personal attributes	Social skills
Awareness of the profession and the Mentor's roles and responsibilities	Adheres to uniform policy
Be aware of own objectives before starting placement	Appreciates teamwork and other people's role
Be motivated	Be friendly, adaptable and co-operate
Bring documentation to placement	Displays respectful and caring behaviour towards patients/relatives at all times
Enthusiastic and interested in the placement area	Good communication skills
Flexible – plans of placement may change	Good social skills – be able to interact with clients/staff in a range of settings
Learn and appreciate the mentor's role on placement	Good time keeper
Open to new learning	Professionalism – in relation to being a student of nursing
Positive attitude and questioning practice	Punctuality and politeness
Self-directed learning at times	Respect the workload and responsibilities that qualified staff have to their workplace
Show initiative and be reliable	Talk to the patient and their family
Get stuck in and involved	Appear and work in a professional manner
Values the placement ethos	Inform mentor if any problems

TABLE 1.3   *The most significant attributes that a mentor possesses*

Health professional	Most important role
1 Nursing mentors	Teacher, supporter and mode
2 Midwifery mentor	Facilitator and teacher
3 Nursing mentee	Teacher and supporter
4 Midwifery mentee	Teacher and supporter
5 Medic mentee	Advisor and supporter

Source: (Bray and Nettleton, 2007)

used more effectively in order to emphasize the importance of self-directed learning in students. The eight domains of mentorship can be focused around three main approaches to supporting the student and helping them gain as much as possible from the practice placement although the facilitation of learning is the one theme throughout (see Box 1.7).

Box 1.7   Three themes throughout the domains of mentorship

1   Facilitation of learning: domains 1, 2, 3, 4, 5, 6, 7, 8.
2   Assessment: domains 3, 4, 8.
3   Creating an environment for learning: domains 1, 3, 5, 6, 7, 8.

(NMC, 2008a)

Therefore, students need to be aware of the importance of taking responsibility for their own learning and capitalizing on the resources that they find more effective. The importance of accessing health information is a priority in contemporary healthcare and although primarily designed for service users, students can also benefit from them as a useful resource.

Bradshaw (2008: 3) states: 'Information and choice are indispensable if we are to achieve a truly patient-centred NHS in which standards and quality are constantly improved.' Healthcare students need to be aware of current changes and how efforts are being made to improve the service for those who need to access it. NHS Choices (2008) is one approach that emphasizes the importance of making the NHS's online service accessible to the public. It is its intention to contribute to achieving better health and well-being by providing appropriate information for patients. The NHS Choices (2008: 5) states: 'The NHS of the future will be one of patient power, patients engaged and taking control over their own health and healthcare.' All healthcare students do need to know and understand how the National Health Service that they intend to work for is changing.

Students need to appreciate that the NHS Choices (2008) has five strategic goals that can affect them, their training and their understanding of the patient's healthcare journey. These goals include:

- *Better access* – using technology to offer a personalized service.
- *Better health* – enabling people to take greater responsibility for their own health and well-being.
- *Better care* – it will help people understand the right treatment and care options for themselves or those for whom they are caring.
- *Better quality through insight* – understanding of the patient, client and carer experience.
- *Better lives* – improving community partnerships to deliver better health.

Mentors need to ensure that their own knowledge is updated in order that they can explain to healthcare students how contemporary changes are influencing their particular nursing speciality. In support, Professor Michael

Thick, Chief Clinical Officer, from the NHS Connecting for Health (2009: 4) states:

> Healthcare is undergoing a paradigm shift, from Industrial Age Medicine to Information Age Healthcare. Information and communication technologies will play a pivotal role in facilitating this change and as these technologies mature and are embedded in clinical practice they will influence future delivery models of healthcare.

Now complete Mentor Activity 1.2 in order to enhance and consolidate your own healthcare awareness.

MENTOR ACTIVITY 1.2

What specific changes nationally and/or locally are happening in your speciality of nursing that will have an impact on the patient's healthcare journey?

Reflect on this question to ensure that your own professional knowledge is updated.

Whatever national or local changes you have identified, there is no doubt that education is an important medium in which to explore, theorize, and implement aspects of care that are intended to improve the patient's healthcare experience. 'During September 2007 Skills for Health issued a consultation on EQuIP, an "Enhancing Quality in Partnership" model for Quality Assurance (QA) of healthcare education, which Skills for Health was commissioned to develop by the Department of Health (DH)' (Skills for Health, 2008: 2). The main philosophy underpinning EQuIP is to examine the quality of healthcare education, and its improvement, as a standardized, and evidence-based model. The associated aims are to do the following:

- Ensure safer, more effective practitioners and service.
- Enhance patient and service user experience of healthcare.
- Reduce QA burden on providers.
- Lead to more responsive and increasingly competent-based education programmes.

There are 11 basic principles that link into an interprofessional education and training programme for healthcare. Mentors will have to enhance their own understanding associated with EQuIP and identify how it relates to their specific healthcare setting. So, within today's NHS there are a number of changes associated with care delivery, communications, education and service management. The mentor needs to ensure that they maintain their knowledge as up to date as possible.

The most significant change in the future will amalgamate all these recommendations in order to improve pre-registration nursing education in their review findings *Nursing: Towards 2015* (NMC, 2008c). This review was in favour of a degree-level minimum nurse training programme, and only awarding a diploma if the student is unable to achieve degree level but is safe and effective in practice. The importance of advocating a degree-minimum training programme was:

- the need for critical thinking skills in an increasingly diverse and complex climate of healthcare delivery and patient needs;
- to bring the UK into line with other countries and with other healthcare professions in the UK.

In the report on consultation findings, the NMC (2008c: 4) states:

> There have been considerable developments in healthcare policy and delivery in recent years, and it is imperative that pre-registration nursing education continues to enable nurses to work safely and effectively to meet the needs of patients now and in the future.

Mentors will need to ensure that they maintain their awareness of what will happen to pre-registration nurse training in the future so that they can ensure that their knowledge remains current.

Mentorship is a dynamic and progressive role that continues to develop according to the health service changes, local healthcare requirements and recommendations from national and statutory bodies – the NMC and the HPC. One of the main roles of mentorship relates to the process of assessment. In order for the evaluation of the assessment to be realistic, the student must be given time with their mentor so that their progress can be discussed and appropriately monitored. Hinchliff (2009) believes that time management is important but this process unfortunately breaks down in the clinical setting due to staff shortages and workload. The length of placement must be deemed long enough in order that an evaluation of learning can be ascertained. The student must be allowed time and access to appropriate resources according to their training programme, speciality, and this will be enhanced if the mentor shows a positive commitment to the student's development.

Summative assessments are used to ascertain the student's ability to deliver specific skills, including communication and interpersonal skills and a variety of healthcare requirements. These assessments are reliable because each student is assessed against a pre-determined checklist, the same criteria is applied to all. These are more challenging because the student has to pass at an agreed level (40–50 per cent) and often there is a limit on the number of attempts that they may take. Mentorship is therefore a rewarding and self-fulfilling component of the healthcare professional repertoire of roles and responsibilities. It is interesting, ever changing but at times extremely challenging.

Frequently asked questions

Mentors

Q. Why do some students fail to show any interest, enthusiasm or motivation whilst working in the practice placement? This is not an unusual situation and it does cause us some concern as mentors.

A. Students' responses to their practice placement may vary according to their perception of what they are supposed to be achieving. For some students the placement may be a non-branch experience and hence their commitment may be reduced or not so apparent. This may be determined by the enthusiasm shown by the mentor to ensuring that the student's experiences are as productive, interesting and meaningful as possible. However, the lack of interest, enthusiasm and motivation may be because the student doesn't appreciate that particular placement, the efforts made by the mentor to enhance their mentorship experience or all the facets of learning that it has to offer. Alternatively, this behaviour may be as a result of previous negative placement experiences and/or 'poor' mentor experience that has left the student sceptical regarding the supportive roles that mentors can offer. Both student and mentor need to value the importance of mentorship and how each other can learn from this professional relationship.

Q. Why do some students lack initiative and have to be told what to do all the time – they seem to lack spontaneity?

A. The reasons why some students appear to lack initiative and spontaneity may be due to their intrapersonal variables – their insecurity, reduced self-esteem and threatened self-efficacy. Mentoring a student who feels this way is a challenge, frustrating but also rewarding if the mentor can initiate a more positive response by encouraging the student to value the placement for all the learning opportunities that are available for them to access. If you continue to have concerns, discuss them with the student, your colleagues (if possible) and possibly the student's own Personal Tutor because you have to feel confident in verifying objectively and constructively that student's achievements in their documentation. The mentor will need to ascertain the student's previous experience of mentorship and, if negative, correct any misconceptions that the student may have.

Students

Q. Why do some mentors make it obvious that they don't want to be a mentor and that the student is an inconvenience or creates added pressure that they could well do without?

A. Mentorship is a two-way supportive relationship between the student and healthcare professional, in which both have to appreciate the other's role. Sometimes students are a little egocentric and tend to forget that mentorship is only one of the many roles that a mentor is trying to juggle and deal with. They have their own commitment to fulfilling their job description which relates to leadership responsibilities, management pressures and facilitating learning as a teacher in the practice setting whilst ultimately trying to deliver nursing care. Sometimes students do need to take a step back, observe their mentor and appreciate that mentorship is an added responsibility but also that within the mentor–student relationship both parties need to value each other.

Q. Why does my mentor insist on calling me 'the student', don't they realize that I have a Christian name and sometimes it is appropriate to call me by it?

A. This is a valid question and one that does concern students throughout their nurse training. Unfortunately, the answer is not an easy one because this response from the mentor may be a professional stance in front of the patient or their family members. There may be a number of other reasons why this happens, so the student does need to be assertive and share their concerns with the mentor in order to achieve a mutual compromise and understanding. The student needs to explain why this ineffective approach to communications and interpersonal skills is so upsetting to them and how they feel that it is devaluing the mentorship process.

Chapter summary

This chapter has examined the process of mentorship pertinent to nursing, midwifery and other health professional students. On completion you have learned about:

- how education has progressed since the introduction of mentorship into the healthcare setting;
- the Nursing and Midwifery Council's (2008a) four-stage developmental framework for mentors;
- the Health Professions Council's (2007b) specific standards of conduct, performance and ethics although both Councils' standards are inter-linked;
- what mentors expect from their students in order to ensure the continuity of effective mentorship;
- how mentorship has three main inter-linking domains: facilitation of learning, assessment and creating an environment for learning.

Further reading

Nursing and Midwifery Council (2008a) *Standards to Support Learning and Assessment in Practice: NMC Standards for Mentors, Practice Teachers and Teachers*, 2nd edn. London: NMC.

This is a vital document which can be obtained from the NMC or downloaded from their website (www.nmc-uk.org). This document introduces a number of contemporary issues associated with mentorship and some of these will be discussed throughout the book. The four stages within the developmental framework are examined and explained effectively.

2

How can the mentor assist the student to become part of the healthcare team?

David Kinnell

Nursing and Midwifery Council (2008a): Eight domains of mentorship
Domain One: Establishing an effective working relationship

Aim

Demonstrate effective relationship building skills sufficient to support learning, as part of a wider interprofessional team, for a range of students in both practice and academic learning environments.

Outcomes

Stage 1: Nurses and Midwives

- Work as a member of the multi-professional team, contributing effectively to team working.
- Support those who are new to the team integrating into practice learning environment.
- Act as a role model for safe and effective practice.
- Develop effective working relationships based on mutual trust and respect.

(Continued)

(Continued)

Stage 2: Mentor

- Demonstrate an understanding of factors that influence how students integrate into practice settings.
- Provide ongoing and constructive support to facilitate transition from one learning environment to another.
- Have effective professional and interprofessional working relationships to support learning for entry to the register.

Introduction

Mentorship is undoubtedly one of the most rewarding components of a qualified healthcare professional's role. Although the demands on and expectations of that role continue to increase within a contemporary healthcare service, and the responsibilities incurred at times seem somewhat overwhelming, mentorship is the feature that will allow the mentor the opportunity to reflect with satisfaction when hopefully the healthcare student endorses their sincere gratitude for all the guidance given. In reality, the feedback from the learner is dependent on their view of how effective the mentor has been in supporting and assessing them throughout their practice placement. Sometimes mentorship is a little problematic and therefore the gratitude from the student may not be so evident. However, reflecting on a collective overview of mentoring experiences, mentors do highlight the positive and worthwhile aspects of their role. In mentor preparation training programmes and then the ongoing continuation of mentor updates and support, the mentor is encouraged to explore the complexity of their role and the valued contribution that they will make or are making to the continuity and development of their specific profession. Mentorship is therefore challenging, rewarding, satisfying, but at times somewhat frustrating. This chapter will explore how mentors can assist healthcare students to establish an effective working relationship. The chapter discusses mentorship domain one (NMC, 2008a).

The mentor's role in team working

This chapter will focus on these NMC (2008a) outcomes in an attempt to help trainee mentors, mentors newly registered on a mentor database and also established mentors to reflect on their role now and in the future. In mentorship there are generic principles that can be applied to nurses, midwives and other allied professions. These generalized principles are then further developed to explore the individual healthcare specialities and their specific professional needs.

These are then amalgamated with the general principles and practices that constitute the practicality of the mentor's role. A supportive link throughout is the awareness and understanding that are encapsulated within the underpinning theoretical perspectives that comprise effective communication and interpersonal skills.

Therefore, within its ever changing remit mentorship can be summarized as:

1   The process of facilitating a healthcare student's learning, ensuring that some of the theoretical concepts incorporated within the psychology of learning have been explored.
2   In order to appreciate the importance of individualistic assessment, it is essential to reflect on the psychosocial influences that will have an impact on the student's behaviour and how their social circumstances are an integral part of who they are.
3   There is a debatable issue surrounding the difference in expectations that healthcare students have regarding their practice-based placements. What constitutes an effective environment may not meet the needs of all students.

Therefore, gaining an awareness of healthcare student individuality may be useful for the mentor when assessing the effectiveness of their student's behaviour within their particular healthcare team. The focus of this chapter will establish the significance of mentorship and its necessity within training programmes for all healthcare students. In order to do this, it is essential to explore the criteria that make an effective healthcare team and the factors that influence that working relationship.

There are a number of intra-personal variables that are significant in understanding human behaviour and why some interactions are not as effective as they could be. A selection of these intra-personal variables will be examined, in a manner that aims to enhance the mentor's understanding of the identified underpinning theoretical perspectives (Moseley and Davies, 2007; Webb and Shakespeare, 2008). However, the intention initially is to apply these theoretical concepts using a generalized focus to the process of mentorship that is applicable to any allied professions that are involved in an interprofessional approach to enhancing student learning.

The intra-personal variables explored include attitudes, emotions, and the self-concept. The aim is to précis the main theoretical concept identified, provide a brief overview and emphasize its significance in understanding the mentor–student relationship. It is anticipated that this will condense previous learning within the social sciences or introduce the topics in order to stimulate further learning as part of mentor training or continued development. The content of this chapter hopefully will be used to complement the theoretical content that has been incorporated into mentor training programmes so it can be used to encourage discussion, critical analysis and/or evaluation of the theory to practice debate.

To help you enhance your understanding of the mentor's role, you need to complete Mentor Activity 2.1, this will show what a healthcare student may expect from their mentor.

MENTOR ACTIVITY 2.1

What are the qualities and skills that make an effective mentor?

Answer this question and make a list. Compare with that at the end of this chapter.

Now you have explored the qualities and skills of an effective mentor, consider Case study 2.1 and reflect on your own experiences. The student involved could be in nursing, midwifery or from the allied professions.

CASE STUDY 2.1

You are mentoring a first-year healthcare student, on his first placement. He does not appear to relate to the patients, and he has ineffective communication skills. When you tell him of your concerns, he becomes very defensive and annoyed that you are expressing these opinions.

He states that he is learning and achieving the expected learning outcomes. Your colleagues also share their concerns about his apparent lack of interest and behaviour.

How would you deal with this situation?

Unfortunately, when mentorship appears to become problematic, it does have an unpleasant effect on the cohesiveness of the working relationship and often if not managed appropriately, can develop into an emotive situation (Moseley and Davies, 2007). How this particular case study should be managed will be viewed differently by mentors according to their own previous experience, the type of mentor training and update undertaken but consider the following suggestions to help you learn from this experience.

Consider the following suggestions:

1 Make sure that the concerns are justified and expressed in an objective manner. Avoid subjectivity and be specific, supporting your concerns with precise examples.
2 Arrange a comfortable room and ensure the timing does not create problems for the practice placement. The need for privacy and time to discuss the concerns is paramount and can influence the result of your discussion.
3 Try to avoid interruptions by ensuring that other staff members realize that they should not disturb you unless really necessary. This will help you and the student to feel more relaxed and see this as a constructive feedback and not a destructive interaction.
4 Consider the main points of your concerns = 'does not relate well to patients':

   (a) Clarify what you mean, why do you feel that this problem exists?
   (b) Identify the specific aspects of the problem and the significance to your patients and the practice placement philosophy of care.
   (c) Allow the student to respond to your concerns and then devise an Action Plan to help him develop his contribution to the team's dynamics as part of his personal and professional development.

5 Consider the point = 'has ineffective communication and interpersonal skills'

   (a) State why you are concerned and how the decision was made.
   (b) Consider the importance of direct and indirect observations from patients, clients, service users, their families and your colleagues.
   (c) However, be careful that this does not appear to be harassment.
   (d) Allow the student time to respond and devise an Action Plan as a way forward.

6 Identify what he has already achieved:

   (a) How many NMC (2004c) outcomes has he achieved and the type of evidence he has collected?
   (b) What level does he think he is working at depending on the specific assessment criteria being used?
   (c) Verify his achievements in his Ongoing Achievement Record (NMC, 2008a), sign and date the outcomes.
   (d) If there are any problems with providing the student with evidence of his achievements, these should be discussed and help offered as appropriate.
   (e) If his achievements are below the required standard, you must explain what he needs to do to improve the quality, possibly show him an example if appropriate.

7 However, you must emphasize that his progress will be monitored and academic support will be sought if required. Initially, although the discussion is written down and documented, the placement manager may want to resolve this locally and only involve the School of Nursing if required.
8 End your discussion on a positive note, emphasizing that the Action Plan devised or amended must be viewed as a positive way forward.

This is only intended to be used as a suggested framework and was the way that this problem was successfully resolved. No doubt from your own reflections or discussion with colleagues you would have generated other ideas, and you need to manage the situation giving negative feedback in a positive way so that it can be seen as constructive and not destructive. You will need to emphasize the student's contribution to the patients' experience of healthcare.

Throughout a patient's healthcare journey they will encounter a number of professionals who are working in partnership in order to ensure that the individual service user's experience meets their perceived expectations. As part of the Medical, Nursing and Allied Health Professions Multi-Disciplinary Team, there are a number of students involved who are observing their mentors deliver the associated aspects of care, according to their healthcare expertise. This interprofessional approach now offers students an understanding and appreciation of each other's roles and responsibilities and how they inter-relate in order to meet the patients' physical, social and psychological needs. Therefore, part of a mentor's role is to assist the student to gain an awareness of what makes an effective healthcare team.

What makes an effective healthcare team?

Whyte (2007) emphasizes the importance of assessing members' individual and collective perspectives on teamwork dynamics. Healthcare students will have a varied contribution to make to team dynamics, depending on their status and the remit of their role. There is a debatable dichotomy between idealism and reality because of the nature of human interaction that mentorship is built upon. Mentorship training programmes usually explore the roles and responsibilities of the mentor and emphasize the valued personal and professional development that this incurs now and in the future. The process of mentorship continues to respond to guidance offered by professional bodies. The Nursing and Midwifery Council (2008a) and the Health Professions Council (2004; 2007a) are both instrumental because they offer suggestions that are pertinent to all nurses, midwives and allied professions.

There will inevitably be marked variations and expectations according to whether the healthcare student is working in a community, a hospital or a voluntary and independent sector placement. Their contribution will be determined by the individuality of the patients, residents or service users and their healthcare needs. As a mentor, it is therefore essential that this individuality is appreciated in order to assist the healthcare student to feel part of the team. It is also necessary to have an awareness of the dichotomy that may exist within the different groups in the healthcare setting and some mentors may find this challenging. However, as your experiences of mentorship develop, so will your appreciation of the individuality of the healthcare student and how you can make a difference and help them develop their knowledge, skills and attitudes whilst being a member of your healthcare team.

Establishing effective working relationships

Intra-personal variables

All mentors would find it useful to explore a number of associated psycho-social variables that could offer an understanding of the individuality expressed by their student. Mentorship is viewed as a positive experience (Myall et al., 2008), students are given the opportunity to work with their ideal role model (Donaldson and Carter, 2005) and the mentor helps the student to develop their skills and confidence (RCN, 2007b). Webb and Shakespeare (2008) explored 'judgements about mentoring relationships in nurse education' focusing on the relationship of both the mentor (Box 2.1) and the student.

Box 2.1 Characteristics of good mentors

- Enthusiasm: For students, good mentors were those who were enthusiastic about their own work and about passing on their knowledge to students.
- Attitudes: Mentor's attitudes towards their students were crucial.
- Being there: Students valued mentors who prepared them for new experiences and then, when they thought that they were ready, stood by while students put what they had been taught into practice. (Webb and Shakespeare, 2008)

From the various research studies the value of the mentor is clearly identified. Now consider Case study 2.2 and reflect on how you would deal with this situation.

CASE STUDY 2.2

A second-year mature student nurse complained to her Personal Tutor about her mentor who she thought was being extremely unpleasant towards her. During the discussion it appeared that the student felt she had been singled out and no matter what she did, it was wrong. This constant negative feedback was difficult to cope with and during her discussion this student became very tearful.

Her concerns centred round the way she was treated as opposed to a male student in her same cohort. Her mentor demanded more evidence before she would verify the proficiencies, as opposed to her colleague. Her colleague was allowed to arrange insight visits associated with the placement. She was not allowed to do this, as her mentor stated that she wanted to work every shift with her, 100 per cent of her time on this placement and she would teach her all she needed to know about this speciality.

There was an obvious personality clash between the two. This arose for various reasons, one possible factor was the differentiation in age; the mentor was much younger than the student. The student felt that her mentor disregarded her life experiences and her previous insight into nursing. As a student she felt de-valued, undermined and that her mentor did not give her any respect for what she was achieving.

The situation went from worse to worse, the School of Nursing was later involved, as was the placement manager. She tried to work with other mentors on the ward but they said that they did not want to get involved. The student was requesting help and wanted to be moved from this placement.

What can you learn from this case study to help you develop your mentorship skills?

Case study 2.2 is clearly a complex situation but it is useful for mentors to gain an awareness of the diversity of their role, in order to differentiate between effective and ineffective mentorship. In this domain the importance of understanding factors that influence how effectively or not students integrate into your practice placement need to be explored. It is anticipated that the discussion in this section will help contribute to your understanding of establishing an effective working relationship with healthcare students. The following intra–personal variables in Box 2.2 will be explored: attitudes, emotions, and the self-concept.

Box 2.2   Intra-personal variables influencing an effective student – mentor working relationship

- attitudes
- emotions
- the self-concept

An understanding of attitudes expressed in the healthcare setting

There are a number of definitions that collectively emphasize that an attitude reflects the way we think (cognitive component), and the way we feel (affective component), representing the internal covert component of who we are. This will subsequently have an influence on the overt behaviour, the external component that is displayed by an individual (see Box 2.3). These components are inter-linked and relate to the *three-component view* highlighted by Rosenberg and Hovland (1960) and described by Gross (2005).

Box 2.3   The components of an attitude

- the way we think – cognitive;
- the way we feel – affective
  = these are the covert aspects of a person and cannot always be seen or measured but the end result that mentors will see is
- the way we behave – the overt behaviour that students display, that may influence the way that they are assessed by their mentors
  = knowledge, skills and professional attitudes.

The cognitive (the way we think)

The cognitive component could help the mentor understand why the healthcare student thinks the way they do. Therefore, it is important that as part of establishing an effective working relationship, the mentor needs to appreciate the level of training the student is currently working at, in order to ascertain the appropriate medical jargon that would help to enhance their learning. It is anticipated that the mentor will assist the student to develop their cognitive awareness and enhance their ability in relating theory to practice, irrespective of the type of healthcare setting (RCN, 2004).

A number of educational resources and strategies could assist the student in developing their knowledge of altered pathophysiology, the aetiology of the patient's condition requiring healthcare interventions, assessment and associated management. The use of theoretical frameworks, models and approaches will help to enhance the cognitive development in healthcare students, irrespective of their specific chosen speciality. The effectiveness of the mentor's support will assist with the healthcare student's understanding of their roles and responsibilities, and, hence, the development of how they feel. There are generic outcomes that can be achieved and are transferable from one healthcare setting to another.

Healthcare students, irrespective of their specific profession, should understand and appreciate the importance of:

- professional autonomy, accountability and boundaries;
- valuing the importance and necessity for confidentiality;
- demonstrating a professional duty of care;
- contributing to the interprofessional team philosophy,
- appreciating each individual's roles and responsibilities within a collaborative approach to healthcare delivery and valuing the feelings of the individual whilst undertaking their individualistic role. (NMC, 2008a; HPC, 2004; 2007a)

The affective (the way we feel)

The affective component will be influenced by the cognitive domain, is subjective and relates to the feelings of an individual. Within a healthcare setting, irrespective of the type of profession, the mentor will have an influence on how the student feels. Mentors work with the full range of students, from the novice to the student who occupies the role as an assistant to the first level nurse. Therefore, the mentor's role will be challenging, frustrating at times, but hopefully rewarding as they help prepare the student to feel that they are prepared to become a qualified professional.

The student will observe their mentor and learn from direct observation by respecting them as a role model, and learning how to deal with their feelings when facing a number of healthcare situations and dilemmas. Watson and Harris (2000) emphasize the significance of having a 'good' role model in the practice setting. A classic statement by Bandura (1965) highlights the fact that people will adopt the standards of behaviour demonstrated by respected models. Forty years later, Donaldson and Carter (2005) reinforced the view that students would like a role model whom they respected and felt that their behaviour was appropriate to emulate. This covert behaviour is represented in the overt behaviour displayed when caring for patients, clients and service users.

The behavioural (the way we behave)

The third component *the behavioural* (or *conative*) could be regarded as the end product of mentorship. When working with their mentor the student will model their professional behaviour and re-enact what has been learnt. The overt behaviour is one of the first assessments that the mentor makes, they must ascertain if the student is safe, has effective communication and interpersonal skills, and how successful they are developing their professional behaviour. The assessment strategy using direct observations is the feedback process of how much the student can follow instructions following demonstration, relating theory to practice (RCN, 2004).

All healthcare students will start their training undertaking a theoretical classroom-based instructional period. When they are undergoing the practice-based experience, it will allow the mentor the opportunity to observe their behaviour and reflect on the significance of their attitude, the way they think, feel and behave and how appropriate it is for their chosen profession. However, Calman et al. (2002) also warn that assessments could actually reflect on how well students did or did not 'fit into' the practice team; this is a consideration that mentors need to be aware of and reflect on.

There are a number of theories and functions related to the concept of attitudes, these are interesting and thought-provoking. They help an understanding of what makes an effective working relationship. They also highlight the important role that the mentor has in shaping the student's attitude and reciprocal mutual trust and respect that have been established in the professional relationship. They represent *intra-personal* (internal, personal and individualistic variables) and *interpersonal* relationships, the discourse between the individual and others that they communicate with. This subsequently has significant implications for both the mentor and the healthcare student; consider these as you complete Mentor Activity 2.2.

MENTOR ACTIVITY 2.2

What variables could influence the healthcare student's development of their professional attitudes?

Reflect on this question before continuing.

When completing Mentor Activity 2.2, you could consider the student's understanding and views on the following:

- the impact of contemporary society;
- the changing image of the healthcare profession;
- society's view of the National Health Service;
- the student's own experiences of being a patient or recipient of healthcare services;
- the impact of the media;
- individuality and service user's responsibility for their health status;
- the cost effectiveness of providing effective healthcare;
- the different stages within the patient's healthcare journey.

This is not an exhaustive list but by reflecting on your own experiences, values and beliefs and that of the student, it will help you to correlate the two in order to understand the importance of establishing an effective working relationship. However, attitudes are influenced and accentuated by emotions that the student is experiencing at that time.

Emotions: helping mentors understand students' behaviour

Clore (1994) describes emotions as mental states and that they are special kinds of feelings. In support, Parkinson (1997: 2) states: 'Emotions imply a certain relationship between a person and some object, person (including the self) or event (real, remembered, or imagined).' In order to try and understand individual differences, some psychologists identify that it is necessary to explore the concept of emotions, their components and functions. Psychological research into emotion focuses on four variables associated expressive behaviour and motivated actions (see Box 2.4). This is a useful checklist for mentors who are trying to understand a student's behaviour.

Box 2.4   Four variables associated with emotional experience

- situational evaluations and interpretations
- bodily changes
- expressive behaviour
- motivated actions

Parkinson (1997) explores situational evaluations and interpretations, emphasizing that different emotions are characterized by different evaluations of the situation. For example, positive emotions, such as happiness and pride, are associated with primary appraisals that the situation is beneficial to personal concerns, whereas negative emotions such as anger, fear and sadness suggest that the situation is being detrimental to the individual. Emotions may be further differentiated on the basis of aspects of secondary appraisal. If the situation is appraised as unfavourable, and coping potential is appraised as low and unlikely to improve, then the emotional state experienced is likely to be depression and sadness.

Throughout their training, healthcare students are exposed to a number of practice-based placements or experiences. The mentor has to remember what it was like when they were a student, and the range of emotions experienced on the various placements. The role of the mentor is to help the student relate theoretical concepts to the practice-based experience that they are undertaking. Some healthcare students will thoroughly enjoy their placement. Not only will they achieve their required practice-based competency, outcome, or proficiency, and relate theory to practice for their written assignments, they will also reflect on their practice experience with a positive stance. Conversely, the interpretation and evaluation of the experience may have negative connotations, and these will be reflected in the student's evaluation of placements if the reason they entered nursing does not actually correlate to the experiences gained during their practice placement (Allan et al., 2008).

The student may feel that they were not welcome in the healthcare team, and that their mentor views them as a burden that they could do without. Students reflect on their feelings at the end of their mentorship experience and criticize the negative, the lack of support they were given. They criticize mentors for their lack of enthusiasm as it appeared that this was a role enforced upon them, and not one that they particularly enjoy undertaking (Myall et al., 2008). It is inevitable that a student experiencing negative subjective interactions will undergo the emotions that they describe as being unfavourable. However, some students are naïve and forget that the mentor's primary responsibility is to care for their patient, client or service user. Mentorship is an extra role that they undertake in association with their management responsibilities but it inevitably has positive rewards, both personally and professionally (Allan et al., 2008). Most mentors in their own evaluation and interpretations do view mentorship as a positive experience.

There appears to be agreement in most psychology books that the following three are the main components of an emotion and this would be useful for the mentors to consider when they are trying to gain an understanding of the behaviour displayed by their healthcare student. The first is pathophysiological responses; the second is subjective expression; and the third is the external behaviour displayed. Pathophysiological responses can be attributed to the sympathetic division of the autonomic nervous system – the response system is partly mediated by an increase in circulating epinephrine from the endocrine system.

The resultant responses influence the following:

- Blood pressure and pulse rate increase.
- Respiration increases.
- The pupils dilate.
- Perspiration increases.
- The secretion of saliva and mucus decreases.
- The blood sugar level increases to provide more energy.
- The hairs on the skin become erect, causing 'goose pimples'. (Gross, 2005)

This list serves as a reminder for mentors to help understand some of the responses that may be identified in students working in any healthcare environment and may represent how safe and secure that they feel. These may also be displayed during the first day on a new placement and it would be advantageous for mentors to reflect on their own training and the emotions that they felt when they were in the same situation.

Both Eysenck (2002) and Gross (2005) describe the subjective emotional component that an individual may present in their facial expression and that is indicative of their affective feelings. There are six primary emotions that it could be argued are universal and representative of all human cultures, despite their diversity. These six emotions are surprise, fear, disgust, anger, happiness and sadness, and because of their commonality, they are innate.

Healthcare students will inevitably share their emotional expressions throughout their allocated placement, what the mentor needs to remember is that the facial expression is an indication of how the student is feeling and, when negative, the need to clarify and discuss in order to resolve any misconception. If there are any signs of disappointment, the mentor needs to clarify why the student may feel this way and review their practice-based experience. This early facial warning signal may prevent the student from feeling disappointed and the student will then transform this negative into a more positive end result.

Some students may feel that they are not achieving what they are supposed to, or in comparison, if they are working with another student of the same status, the disappointment may be because their colleague is being given all the learning opportunities to develop and achieve. In some cases, students will not verbally express these feelings but may find it difficult not to display them in their subjective expression.

It is useful for the mentor to reflect on the components of emotions as the theoretical concepts can offer an explanation of why some healthcare students appear to behave the way that they do. Mentors may label the student as not being interested, that they have no motivation, and they lack enthusiasm. This inappropriate negative labelling may be as a result of not interpreting the student's emotional signals or may be as a result of perceptual distortion. Students could argue that they tried to fit into the team, and hence be an effective team member but for whatever reason, no matter what behaviour they displayed, it was not valued in a positive manner. This misconception could have serious implications when the mentor is assessing which competencies, outcomes or proficiencies the healthcare student has or has not achieved. Now read Case study 2.3 for an example of positive mentorship.

CASE STUDY 2.3

A first-year student recently reflected on her first placement and subsequently her first experience of mentorship. She was impressed and extremely surprised by the success and support that she gained from working with her mentor, who made her feel part of the ward team.

This was her first healthcare experience and the mentor respected her and the contribution that she apparently made to the team. Despite the age difference, this younger mentor had valued her as an individual and helped her to develop her knowledge and skills appropriately. The student felt this mentor truly respected her for the person that she was.

What can you learn from this experience?

The significance of understanding the self-concept and its importance to the mentorship process

The success of the mentor and student relationship is dependent on each person understanding and respecting the other. In order to enhance the effectiveness it is important to reflect on what makes us the person that we are (see Box 2.5). However, different authors do tend to vary in their interpretation of what is meant by the self-concept although merely being aware of this could be advantageous for mentors when understanding some student's behaviour.

Box 2.5   The self-concept

The self-concept capitalizes on intra-personal variables of attitudes and emotions, and comprises:

- the self-image
- self-esteem
- the ideal self

(Gross, 2005)

The self-image offers an explanation of the way we describe ourselves, focusing on two categories: social roles and personality traits. It is important for mentors to appreciate the social roles that the student may have – partner, parent, unpaid carer – because this may have an impact on their behaviour when on placement. It is anticipated that students have evaluated how they intend to juggle their many social roles as well as trying to complete their specific healthcare training. Hopefully this has been discussed before they start their training programme. However, the student's social circumstances may change and this will have an influence on their ability to achieve what they would like to.

Gross (2005: 731) describes personality as 'those relatively stable and enduring aspects of individuals which distinguish them from other people, making them unique, but which at the same time allow people to be compared with each other'. Self-image refers to the personality characteristics or traits that we have. However, it could be argued that there may be a marked difference between what we think we are like and how this may be different from the way other people see us. This second approach to understanding the self-image is a matter of opinion and judgement and is an important consideration when related to mentorship.

The mentor may not realize that they appear in the eyes of the student to be unsupportive, unresponsive, or failing to take their role seriously. Conversely, there is a misconception by the mentor as they might not fully appreciate the efforts, determination, dedication and enthusiasm displayed by the student. This breakdown in effective communication could result in the student not being assessed effectively and hence not being given the recognition they deserve. This is a criticism that some students attribute to their mentors although on reflection, variables such as time constraints and a clash of personality will have a major impact.

The concept of self-esteem has been explored by a number of psychologists such as Gross (2005) and Eysenck (2002), and refers to the emotional state of how good we feel about ourselves. The mentor has a significant role to play in helping healthcare students develop their self-esteem by involving them as much as possible in caring for patients, residents or service users, according to their training programme and professional status. This is particularly significant if mentoring the novice healthcare student because the mentor can be extremely instrumental in influencing that person's self-concept. Most students are conscientious and willing to learn. The skills they undertake will depend on their profession but as soon as the mentor involves the student in interpreting patient's care plans, identifying their role and contribution within the interprofessional team approach, the sooner their self-esteem will develop.

Self-efficacy: confidence building

One of the most significant roles that the mentor undertakes is to help the student develop and establish their confidence whilst appreciating the limitations of their skills. Irrespective of their status, all nursing, midwifery and allied professions students rely on their mentor for this guidance within the respective healthcare settings. The positive development of self-efficacy is a process of helping students develop their confidence and marks the transition from novice, at the start of training, to the expert who is ready for qualification, and subsequent fitness for practice and fitness for award.

Self-efficacy is progressive throughout each student's training and coincides with how they actually feel on practice-based placements. This is problematic on some programmes because of the time duration that in some cases is very brief. Regarded as an insight visit, placement awareness or part of a clinical pathway, some students will only spend a few days or weeks in one area. During that time they will have to gain an understanding of that speciality and its contribution to the patient's healthcare journey. From a self-efficacy perspective, some students do complain that the lack of time does not always allow them the opportunity to take full advantage of what the mentor has to offer. Levett-Jones and Lathlean (2008) explore the importance of 'belongingness', a feeling that students need whilst in their practice placements.

As the healthcare student nears the end of their final year, self-efficacy takes on a different stance as the individual develops their awareness and understanding of what the roles and responsibilities will be when they are qualified. This relates to the difference in accountability from being student status to that as a professional registered with a national organization. The senior students have to complete the required written assignments according to whether they are completing a diploma or degree programme as well as developing their knowledge, skills and attitudes that will be expected from them once registered. One of the main roles in this transition will be their contribution to maintaining an effective working relationship and contributing to both group dynamics and group cohesion.

Once qualified, the students will require the need to review their contribution as a professional, manager and teacher, and how this will impact on their students in the future. Hence, mentorship is an important inherent component of all qualified healthcare professionals in order to ensure the continuity of the individual professions, for all nurses, midwives and allied professions. Also, all lecturers in higher education institutes should have a commitment to mentorship, therefore appreciate mentor preparation training in both pre-registration diploma and degree programmes. They should also have an awareness of the delivery of post-registration mentor training programmes, mentor updates and mentor support. This diversity should allow the opportunity to value mentorship from both perspectives and to feed back to both parties – supporting both students and mentors. An awareness of the self-concept serves to stimulate a discussion of why mentorship can work so effectively.

However, exploring the underpinning theoretical perspectives associated with intrapersonal variables does offer some suggestions or an

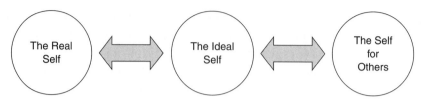

FIGURE 2.1   *Three-dimensional model of the self*
Source: (Rogers, 1951).

understanding of the complexities associated with mentorship. A number of models of the self-concept all offer an interesting insight into this approach but it is the classic model proposed by Rogers (1951) that is thought-provoking and offers a simplistic explanation of the individual's behaviour.

There are three aspects to each individual that constitutes to the concept of the self: the real self, ideal self and the self for others. These three inter-related dimensions offer an explanation of what contributes to human behaviour, and although initially introduced by Rogers (1951), still offers an interesting focus for discussion that can be related to the process of mentorship (Figure 2.1).

The *real self* is that part of an individual that relates to their personal inner thoughts and feelings that the person may have and not share with anyone else, even their closest partners or friends. It relates to our internalized psychological functioning and is representative of the person that we really feel ourselves to be. This first component relates to the personal attributes that we feel that we have and is indicative of the unique characteristics and qualities that makes us who we are – the idiographic approach of our personality. Working with mentors, there is no doubt that they do try to ensure that the healthcare student's practice-based experience is beneficial and contributes to their continued progress. However, as a result of the real self, then maybe this offers an explanation of why mentors fail to 'really get to know the student' and why some students fail to discuss with their mentors why they don't feel that they are achieving what they hoped to achieve. This complexity of human nature constitutes a discussion point but fails to offer a solution to enhancing effective working relationships.

In contrast, the *ideal self* represents the person that we would like to be. This component therefore is reflective of our hopes, aspirations and the ambitions that we have for our future. Whilst working with healthcare students, this is one aspect of their self-concept that the mentor is influential in helping them to develop. On arrival in the practice setting, the healthcare student will be encouraged to share with their mentor what it is that they hope to achieve during their allocated time. The mentor's role is to discuss with the student their expectations and the feasibility of actually achieving what it is they expect to achieve.

Once this has been clarified, it does allow the mentor the opportunity to encourage the student to develop an action plan to ensure that their idealism becomes a reality. If this works effectively, then it is one of the most positive attributes of mentorship. However, mentors report that some students are not aware of what it is that they have to actually accomplish, despite the fact that they may have written practice-based assignments to complete. In association with this, knowledge, skills and attitudes have to be developed and students should be aware of which relevant competencies, outcomes or proficiencies they have to achieve, and the mentor has to sign to verify that accomplishment.

According to Rogers (1951), the final component of the self, is the *self for others* which represents the way we present ourselves to the outside world. This is the façade that we often hide behind and it could be argued that it does not always represent how we truly think and feel. In order to become part of an effective team it may be necessary to conform and appear to be the person that other people want us to be, rather than the person that we truly are.

This creates a dichotomy that can have an influence on our contribution to the healthcare team and a concept that mentors need to be aware of. Some healthcare students may present themselves to various team staff in a different manner, which may contrast with how they present themselves to their mentor. The student will view the mentor as the person who has the ultimate responsibility to verify and sign what the student has achieved, and more importantly, what they have failed to achieve.

These three components overlap and comprise the condition of being congruent or harmonious with our self-concept. The way we perceive ourselves, the way we want to be seen and the way that others perceive us, are all influential in formulating a congruent state. However, if the student is not 'happy' or 'contented' with one of their three components, it can lead to the state of being incongruent or disharmonious. This situation may be caused if the student is unhappy on placement, is not contented with the image that they are portraying to the healthcare team or feel that they are not achieving what they should be and this could lead them to being incongruent.

The mentor must therefore consider the significance of this theoretical concept, discuss with the student the potential of its significance and once an area of concern has been identified, then this negative experience could be converted to a more positive healthy situation. However, dealing with subjective expression can be difficult because of the emotions that are displayed, and the personality of the individuals involved. Whichever approach to mentorship is adopted, mentors of nursing and midwifery students, as well as other allied professions could benefit from reflecting on the intra-personal variables that may have an impact on the way healthcare students think, feel and behave. Mentors do endeavour to undertake their role as effectively as possible and in accordance with the NMC (2008a; 2008b) and the requirements identified by the RCN (2007b) and the HPC (2007b; 2008).

What qualities and skills make an effective mentor?

A number of third-year student nurses (2003–2008) were asked this question in their final management semester, as part of a classroom activity. These students were all asked the same question, and encouraged to write down comments that were collated and explored within the classroom. They had all completed 30 months of nurse training and represented the four nursing branches: adult, child, learning disabilities and mental health. Their valued comments have since been used to initiate discussion as part of the mentor training programme and mentor updates.

Box 2.6 is a summary of their comments – compare them with yours in Mentor Activity 2.1.

Box 2.6   Qualities and skills of an effective mentor

Accommodating.
Appreciates the student's knowledge.
Approachable.
Assists student in problem solving.
Awareness of student's limitations.
Being aware of student's learning objectives.
Confident.
Does not refer to the student as the 'student'.
Encouraging and supportive.
Facilitates student's learning.
Flexible – having time to spend with students.
Gives positive feedback to students.
Good communication skills.
Good knowledge of branch of nursing.
Good flexible teaching skills dependent on what level the student is at.
Good negotiator.

Impartial but fair.
Non-judgemental.
Offers constructive criticism in a professional manner.
Patient.
Takes role of mentorship seriously.
Understanding.
Up-to-date knowledge of nurse training programme and documentation.
Values students as individuals.
Wants to be a mentor and is well organized.

This list shows some similarity with other research studies (Myall et al., 2008; Webb and Shakespeare, 2008) and offers a reminder to mentors of what students appreciate when they first enter a new practice placement.

Throughout this chapter the focus has been to encourage all mentors, including those of student nurses, to consider the importance of understanding the factors that influence students whilst they are working as a temporary member of the healthcare team. It is important to remember that all healthcare students should be given ongoing and constructive support throughout their practice placement.

The Nursing and Midwifery Council (2008a) and the Health Professions Council (2004; 2007a–g) are both advocates of interprofessional learning and allied professions working together to contribute to the successful experience of patients throughout their healthcare journey. It is hoped that by exploring the significance of intra-personal variables that all mentors will adopt a more supportive role for the student that they are mentoring.

By exploring the variables that make the 'person' the individual that they are, it hopefully will encourage a more thought-provoking discussion when mentors are comparing their healthcare student with their colleagues. Mentorship is undoubtedly a challenging but nevertheless worthwhile component of all healthcare professionals' roles and responsibilities.

Frequently asked questions

Mentors

Q. Why is my student not as good as the student that my colleague is currently working with? She is much more enthusiastic, ambitious

(Continued)

(Continued)

and eager to learn than my student and she shows a positive approach to being a team member.

A. Each student is an individual and depending on how well they are made to feel in the practice placement, they will respond differently. Domain one focuses on establishing an effective working relationship, you need to ask yourself how successful have you been in achieving the associated mentor outcomes. Students will respond to how they are made to feel.

Q. I just cannot get on with my student. No matter what I do to help him, he appears to be arrogant and condescending. I have tried really hard to help him adapt from his previous practice placement. What am I doing wrong?

A. This chapter has examined a number of individual variables that make each human being different from one another, and hence, the individuality shown by some students. However, the importance of this situation is that ideally each student will have a main mentor as well as a co-mentor. Therefore, you should be able to get support from each other or discuss with your manager regarding the possibility of changing your student.

Students

Q. I have not met my mentor yet and this is my second week in this practice placement. What am I supposed to do?

A. Ideally you should meet your mentor on day one but certainly by the end of the first week in order for them to complete your Orientation and Initial Interview. You must find out if you have an allocated associate/co-mentor and discuss with them your concerns. If not, you will need to contact the placement manager or the Educational Link if possible.

Q. I don't like my practice placement, I feel like I am treated as a 'pair of hands'. I don't seem to be learning anything as I hardly ever see my mentor because they are always in charge of the ward. What should I do?

A. You must tell your mentor or associate/co-mentor how you feel. It is difficult when your main mentor is in charge during a shift but if it is a regular problem, you must express your concerns. It is difficult for mentors to balance all the roles and responsibilities that they have, but mentorship is part of their professional role. You will have to speak to the placement manager or educational link in order to help resolve this issue.

Chapter summary

This chapter has examined how effective mentorship can contribute to helping students become part of the healthcare team. Having completed this chapter, you have learned:

- which factors contribute to make an effective healthcare team in order to enhance the patient's healthcare journey;
- which qualities and skills make an effective mentor in contemporary healthcare;
- the impact that intra-personal variables including attitudes, emotions and the self-concept can have on group cohesion;
- the importance of understanding individual students and why they behave the way they do in the practice setting;
- the complexities that may influence establishing effective working relationships.

Further reading

Donaldson, J.H. and Carter, D. (2005) 'The value of role modelling: perceptions of under-graduate and diploma nursing (adult) students', *Nurse Education in Practice,* 5: 353–9.

This is an interesting research-based article that focuses on the stated topic. This will be valuable for further reading as it extends the discussion regarding the importance of role models and how they enhance the quality of the practice setting.

Gross, R. (2005) *Psychology: The Science of Mind and Behaviour,* 5th edn. London: Hodder Arnold.

Chapter 24: Attitudes and Attitude Change is an extremely useful chapter that explores the topic of attitudes and a number of related issues that will enhance the mentor's understanding of this intra-personal variable.

Royal College of Nursing (2004) *Helping Students Get the Best from their Practice Placements: A Royal College of Nursing Toolkit.* London: RCN.

This is a helpful document for both mentors and healthcare students because it provides a number of checklists on pp. H 10–16 that can help the reader reflect on the effec-tiveness of establishing interprofessional working relationships in the practice setting.

3

Facilitating the learning of healthcare students

David Kinnell
Philip Hughes

Nursing and Midwifery Council (2008a): Eight domains of mentorship
Domain Two: Facilitation of learning

Aim

To facilitate learning for a range of students, within a particular area of practice where appropriate, encouraging self-management of learning opportunities and providing support to maximize individual potential.

Outcomes

Stage 1: Nurses and Midwives

- Co-operate with those who have defined support roles contributing towards the provision of effective learning experiences.
- Share their knowledge and skills to enable others to learn in practice settings.

Stage 2: Mentor

- Use knowledge of the student's stage of learning to select appropriate learning opportunities to meet individual needs.
- Facilitate the selection of appropriate learning strategies to integrate learning from practice and academic experiences.
- Support students in critically reflecting upon their learning experiences in order to enhance future learning.

Introduction

One of the most rewarding aspects of mentorship is being involved in the process of facilitation of learning and being able to share the interest and enthusiasm that you have regarding your health professional role and the speciality of healthcare that you are involved with. The NMC (2008b) and the HPC (2008) highlight the importance of sharing your knowledge and expertise with others. This chapter discusses domain two (NMC, 2008a) and the content is divided into five sections:

- The healthcare learner
- Approaches to teaching or teaching styles
- Theories of learning
- Educational taxonomies
- Teaching styles used in the practice placement.

Following the emphasis and importance placed on the quality and consistency of learning in the clinical environment, the development and learning of the individual learner are key to the healthcare professions. In this way a number of key aspects will be considered when facilitating learning, and also to appreciate how an individual learns, taking into consideration theories from the past.

Facilitation of learning in healthcare

There is no doubt that all professionals can be involved in the facilitation of learning of the healthcare students they work with. Although the process may vary from direct observations, discussions, spontaneous questioning, micro-teaching to more involved semi-structured teaching sessions, all mentors will have their own stance, enthusiasm, motivation and dedication to assist students' progress, and show that practice placement is advantageous to their learning.

The healthcare learner

Mentors need to appreciate the importance of understanding the healthcare student and the potential individual needs that they have, that can influence the effectiveness of the mentorship relationship (Levett-Jones and Lathlean, 2008) – see Box 3.1.

Box 3.1   Understanding the healthcare student

- The level of the learner within their training programme.
- The age of the learner, valuing their appropriate life skill experiences.
- The number of learners who are working at the same time on placement.
- Staff resources and time to spend supporting the individual learner.

Finding out how a person learns is the key to successful teaching and facilitating learning. This particular area should not be underestimated as it requires thought, insight, and a good clinical background. The mentor needs to ensure that they have a clear understanding of the student's training programme and curriculum, and can clarify that this is maintained up to date. Nurse education changes in response to NMC recommendations, and the mentor must appreciate the need for these changes. This area is also quite complex and therefore should not be taken for granted. It is easy to assume that just because one is knowledgeable or an expert in a particular way, then this makes one a good teacher. This may be viewed as a misconception because facilitating learning is an art in itself.

Now complete Mentor Activity 3.1 and reflect on your professional experiences of facilitating learning for healthcare students.

MENTOR ACTIVITY 3.1

How can a mentor ensure that a student nurse or midwife is safe to administer an intramuscular injection?

Answer this question and reflect on your response.

(A similar common or core question could be asked according to your healthcare speciality or profession.)

This response will then generate further questions such as:

- What stage or level of training is the student at?
- Do they have previous knowledge or experience?
- What is the prescribed medicine for injection?
- What type of patient do we have: child, adult, older person, someone with a learning disability or mental health problem?

TABLE 3.1   *Assessing the students' knowledge, skills and attitude – practical skill*

1   Knowledge

- Understanding of the Health and Safety at Work Act (Health and Safety Executive, 1974).
- A working knowledge of the equipment that will be required and an understanding of how to set that equipment up depending on the drug being administered.
- Knowledge of the medication to be given – the reason for giving it and its action.
- Knowledge of anatomy and physiology of the various injection sites, the muscles involved and potential areas of concerns.

2   Skill

- Ability to safely read a drug prescription chart, and to calculate the prescribed medication.
- Demonstrate the correct procedure according to local policy with regard to administering intramuscular injections.
- Demonstrates the correct and safe disposal of the used equipment.

3   Attitude

- Demonstrate effective communication and interpersonal skills associated with your client group for successful administration of the medicine.
- Appreciate the importance of the law and relevant professional code, in order to obtain consent prior to administration of the prescribed medicine.
- Advocate the importance of correct completion of documentation after administration (NMC, 2008d, Standard Eight: Standards for practice of administration of medicines).

Try not to take for granted the skills and understanding that are required to pass this knowledge on. When looking at your own common or core skills, it is important to consider the underpinning theoretical perspectives associated with skill assessment. Consider Table 3.1 and compare with your answer to Mentor Activity 3.1. In order to administer an intramuscular injection safely, it is important to consider the student's knowledge, skills and attitude (NMC, 2004c).

How long will this take to teach the student nurse or midwife? It may take longer than you first thought and yet it is something that many of us do every day (or such skilled procedures associated with your own professional activities). We cope with this by breaking the component parts into more manageable chunks that could formulate a procedural framework. This way we can time the input that is required and the opportunities that can be recognized and employed. The effectiveness of learning any procedure will be influenced by the student's ability to undertake self-directed learning as they can read the NMC guidelines, local policy and procedure manual and nursing text books that explain how the procedure should be safely administered. They will also learn from experiential learning involvement particularly by practising injection technique on a sample of sponge or foam that represents skin, alternatively an orange or other substitute can be used.

Now reflect on your own professional experiences and complete Mentor Activity 3.2.

MENTOR ACTIVITY 3.2

How would you use a range of resources to ensure that students develop appropriate knowledge, skills and attitudes across a range of healthcare skills?

Answer this question and reflect on your response.

So what information do we require in order to make a learning experience useful and worthwhile? There are certain aspects that will help to achieve a good teaching/learning experience if we can consider them or at least take them into account.

Level of learner

What is the level of the student's training?

- Are they first, second, third or fourth year?
- Are they pre-registration or post-registration?

The significance of this is that it will dictate the mentor's expectations, although there may be a problem of taking the student for granted or forming a negative stereotype about them. The mentor must ascertain the student's previous experiences and review these in order to further develop them. The level of the learner may also dictate the use of grammar and language and depth that you might choose on the given subject. With the wide and varied programmes of curricula, then it might be useful to enquire regarding their previous clinical experience. This may be particularly useful with pre-registration students who have been in a support role or that of an assisting role in their chosen branch. At the same time it can be difficult not to take too much for granted, remember that they are students and therefore have a different role to execute.

Age of learner

Many people bring with them life skills to a greater or lesser degree. It would be most unfortunate and a potential disadvantage if the mentor did not explore these attributes. When mentors do this, it can show the value of that person, give them confidence and motivation. The student may have first-hand experience of a particular subject, illness or procedure from a patient or a carer's point of view and be able to offer another angle and therefore add another dimension or perspective.

Number of learners

Many clinical placements have a multiplicity of learners at any given time. This can include different levels of learner from different learning establishments on the same or similar professional pathway, or other professionals, not excluding those students on a post-registration programme or module. This can be an overwhelming time for mentors and resources and requires thought for staff as well as students. Facilitating learning in this way requires balance and this can be difficult given the demands of clinical practice in the twenty-first century. A mentor cannot be all things to all people all of the time. The work load of the student should be carefully considered and distributed among staff, hence the importance of the main mentor who is supported by an associate or co-mentor.

Motivation

Finally, learning is reliant on the student themselves and how much they want to learn. There are a number of motivational theories to consider in order to understand the psychological aspects of drives to learning. Abraham Maslow (1954) looked at the 'Hierarchy of needs'. In this theory he considers that in order to achieve, certain elements in one's life should be in place. Without these elements, then depending upon where you are in the range will be proportional to the inhibition to learning. Some theories point to the need for motivation and suggest that this is a factor in itself. Also for some there is a need to achieve because of a fear of failure. However, Wiener's (1979) theory of motivation emphasizes an individual's search for understanding.

From these points it is apparent that adult learning, in whatever context, should be a shared responsibility and the role of the mentor in helping to facilitate learning should be to make aware or try to understand the student's learning style and to adopt their approach accordingly. Over many years the style generally of teaching has changed.

Approaches to teaching or teaching styles

Two generally recognized opposing styles can be compared. One approach entails a strict teacher who is very much in charge, and who perhaps appears to demonstrate certain corporal or regimented principles. This in some ways could be seen as a pedagogical approach as opposed to the more modern approach of andragogy.

Pedagogy verses andragogy

Pedagogy is derived from two Greek words, 'pais' meaning 'boy' and 'agogos' meaning 'to lead'. As you might assume, the teacher takes control and leads the child in the learning process. The learner could be said to be dependent and is reliant upon the teacher, his approach, attitude and experience. The maturity and motivation and ability are not necessarily considered. The subject or matter is directed and prescribed and its conclusion is anticipated. There may be other outside influencing factors and pressures that might affect learning. The teacher or facilitator has a didactic, instructional or dictatorial approach.

Andragogy is a much later term that was identified by Knowles (1984; 1994) and, in congruence with proposers such as Rogers (1969) and Maslow (1970), puts the student at the centre of the teaching episode. Maslow advocates the importance of learning and that consideration of what is going on in one's life can affect learning and Rogers firmly believes that each individual is unique and has in themselves an innate ability to achieve to the best of their ability and that they can, given the opportunity and guidance, achieve to their highest level.

This is, of course, an opposing viewpoint to pedagogy. It is guiding and self-directing from the learner's viewpoint. There is an appreciation that the student brings with them previous experience, especially adults who have held or performed a different role in the past. It is accepted that because the student is there that they have motivation either internally or externally or both. There is a focus on the student, with negotiation of learning and learning strategies with the student taking equal responsibility for the learning process and outcomes.

Staff resource and time

The NMC (2008a) has recognized that the role of mentor should have a time allowance in order that both Stage One and Stage Two mentors can contribute in accordance with their associated domain two outcomes. The HPC (2008) also emphasizes the importance of all allied health professionals keeping their professional knowledge and skills up to date in order that they can work safely and effectively. Healthcare students will spend time with nursing, midwifery and allied professions whilst gaining an awareness of the patient's healthcare journey and the importance of the interprofessional approach involving a range of different health professions. The NMC (2008a) state that a student should spend at least 40% of their placement time with a mentor.

Theories of learning

There are three basic approaches to understanding the psychology of learning:

- the cognitive approach (covert);
- the humanistic approach (covert);
- the behaviourist approach (overt).

The cognitive approach – cognitivism

This theory explores the concept of understanding the way we think. A number of noted psychologists have contributed to establishing this epistemology from Sigmund Freud (1923), to later theorists including Jean Piaget (1963). It would be useful for mentors to reflect on their previous knowledge of psychology applied to healthcare and update as required by reading an appropriate text (Gross, 2005; Hayes, 2005). Certainly, Piaget is acknowledged for his contribution to understanding the development of the process of thinking in children (see Box 3.2).

Box 3.2   Piaget's four stages of cognitive development

- Sensory motor (birth to 2 years)
- Pre-operational (2–7 years)
- Concrete operational (7–11 years)
- Formal operational (12 years onwards)

If you are caring for children and a healthcare student is involved in that specialist area of care, this structural approach may offer something to help you as a mentor to explain a child's behaviour to that student. Piaget identified that in the sensory-motor stage the child is developing a number of schemas or rules which it will need to understand to enhance its development. The pre-operational stage is when children are learning the importance of mass, length, volume and numbers but because of their egocentrism, this can be problematic. The mentor needs to explain to the healthcare student that the child expects adults to see the world through their eyes and hence care must be taken when using medical jargon. In the concrete-operational stage the child is managing to deal and understand mathematics but healthcare professionals still need to exercise caution to ensure that the child's healthcare journey is not a negative one if this can be avoided. Students may have discussed child development at some time in their career and the mentor will hopefully relate the underpinning theories to a healthcare context.

However, there a number of other contributions to understanding the process of cognitivism, this includes the theory associated with learning styles. Honey and Mumford (1989) explored an individual's style of learning and devised an extensive questionnaire or inventory of 80 questions to identify a person's predominant approach. The scores identified in the inventory suggest that a person might belong to one or several categories (Box 3.3). As you read through the descriptors, relate them to your own learning style and consider what you can do to adapt your practice-based learning strategies to incorporate the healthcare student's individuality.

Box 3.3   Four learning styles

- Activists
- Reflectors
- Theorists
- Pragmatists

Activists are generally well motivated and open to new experiences. They enjoy the here and now and are happy to be immersed in new experiences. They have a tendency to be open-minded, without bias and enthusiastic. Their motto could be 'I'll try anything once' and so can be accused sometimes of rushing in before planning or giving due consideration to the consequences of their actions. Activists are as the title suggests, very active. They enjoy the here and now and therefore brainstorming. However, as soon as the excitement fades, they explore new experiences on which they thrive. They are not finishers or pay attention to fine detail. Activists can be gregarious (fond of people) and therefore the life and soul of a party.

Reflectors like to stand back and ponder on experiences and observe from many different perspectives. They like to collect information or data for themselves or others and then come to a conclusion or opinion. In the process of collection of data, time elapses and so reaching a definitive conclusion can take time. Their personality traits are thoughtfulness and being good listeners, but when they act, they consider the 'whole picture'. Healthcare students are encouraged to develop and use a holistic approach to delivering patient care and hence view a tripartite framework to understand the patient including physical, social and psychological variables.

Theorists adapt and integrate observations, complex but logically sound theories. Their thought processes mean that they think through in a logical manner. They have a tendency to be a perfectionist who won't give up until things fit into a rational scheme. They like logic, rationality and are analytical. They can therefore be a bit rigid in their thinking and feel uncomfortable with subjective judgements, lateral thinking and anything 'flippant'.

Pragmatists are essentially a practical type of person, 'down to earth' who likes to deal with and solve problems. They question if there can be a better way. They like to try out new ideas and to experiment with applications. They can be a little impatient as they like to get on with things. It is anticipated that healthcare students should be pragmatic as whilst in the practice placement they should be developing their skills and applying underpinning theoretical concepts to the direct delivery patient care.

For those who complete the inventory, it may indicate that one style is more prevalent than the other three or usually there is a combination of all four, depending on how the person answers the questions. The main lesson to learn for mentors is that each healthcare student learns in a different way, the learning styles may offer something for you to consider when you are involved in facilitating your student's learning.

The humanistic approach – humanism

Humanism concentrates on the way we feel. Proponents of the theory include Abraham Maslow (1970) and Carl Rogers (1969). The basic belief is that there is real faith in an individual in that they have worth and a fundamental desire to achieve the best that they can for themselves, attaining self-realization through reason and rational thought. Humanism emerged in the 1950s as a reaction by clinical psychologists, social workers and counsellors against behaviourism and psychoanalysis. Humanists believe that each person is unique and individual and possesses capacities not found in other animals. They give priority to the study of human needs and interests. They study the person as a whole and over their life span – self-motivation and goal-setting are of special interest. The humanist style as a teacher is to be a facilitator. The view of the learning process is that it is a personal act to fulfil one's own potential. They look at the cognitive and affective (attitudinal and covert) processes so that a person can achieve self-actualization or self-fulfilment.

Maslow's 'Hierarchy of needs' theory is much used and adopted in psychological nursing as well as educational arenas. It may have a significant historical inception but Maslow is still of importance in understanding how people learn and what can affect their learning process. The fundamental concept is depicted in a diagrammatic format of a triangle, the ideology being that the baseline needs must be met before moving up to the next levels.

This theoretical concept can be applied to patients as is usual in a pre-registration training programme but, from a mentor's perspective, it also offers some considerations. The mentor should be able to conceptualize what it means for the healthcare student when starting a new practice placement. It is hoped that mentors will consider the seven stages identified by Maslow and ensure that these are considered throughout the student's placement and in particular, if the student does not appear to be settling and developing. Consider Maslow's theory (see Box 3.4) and try to use it as a means of generating discussion with the student.

Box 3.4   Maslow's hierarchy of needs

7 **Self-actualization:** realizing one's full potential, 'becoming everything one is capable of becoming'.

6 **Aesthetic needs:** beauty – in art and nature – symmetry, balance, order, form.

5 **Cognitive needs:** Knowledge and understanding, curiosity, exploration, need for meaning and predictability.

4 **Esteem needs:** The esteem and respect of others, and self-esteem and self-respect. A sense of competence.

3 **Love and belongingness:** Receiving and giving love, affection, trust and acceptance. Affiliating, being part of a group (family, friends, work).

2 **Safety needs:** Protection from potentially dangerous objects or situations, (the elements, physical illness). The threat is both physical and psychological (fear of the unknown). Importance of routine and familiarity.

1 **Physiological needs:** food, drink, temperature regulation, elimination, rest, activity, sex. (Start here at the bottom and work upwards).

In contrast, Carl Rogers (1983) was an advocate of humanism focusing on a student-centred approach. Rogers' background was originally in the priesthood, which may have reflected his philosophical approach to learning. His background was entrenched in child and behavioural psychology and he later developed guides and strategies for counselling. He is less mechanistic than some other theorists and explores the qualities of individuals, including both the teacher or mentor and the student. He believed that people have their own potential and qualities to achieve according to their maximum ability and that the teacher is there to support and guide.

From the mentor's perspective, cognitivism is related to how effective information is presented to the healthcare student in order that they can understand, question and ultimately assimilate it. In association, the humanism is the feelings that the mentor helps to generate within their student: the confidence, enthusiasm and self-efficacy. These two components contribute to covert learning; the end product is portrayed in the overt behaviour displayed and witnessed as the mentor directly observes the student within the practice placement.

The behaviourist approach – behaviourism

A group of psychologists have studied human behaviour and propose the theory of behaviourism. This theory looks at overt behaviour from a learning episode. There are a number of well-known theorists, possibly the best-known is Pavlov (1927). Pavlov produced much of his work in the late nineteenth and early twentieth century, experimenting on a stimulus response in dogs. The method was one of association in that food was shown to the dog and a bell rung at the same time to which the dog salivated in anticipation of eating the food. Eventually only the bell itself was rung and the dog still salivated. Unfortunately this type of experimentation is questionable in its methods by today's standards and would suggest that automatic responses are exactly the same in humans.

Moving on to 1938, Skinner looked at classical and operant conditioning. These experiments were carried out with pigeons or mice but the resultant principles can be applied to the process of learning in the practice placement. Classical conditioning is based on the idea of stimulus and response. The reinforcement could unfortunately be negative and hence does not achieve the desired affect. This relates to the way a mentor gives the student negative feedback. The process should be a positive learning experience if the student is to view the comments as constructive. Now read the situation that a first-year student relayed on their return from a hospital ward placement as recorded in Case study 3.1.

CASE STUDY 3.1

Whilst on my last placement a Staff Nurse started shouting my name down the ward. She eventually told me that she wanted to speak to me 'now!' I was concerned because I didn't know what I had done but the situation was made worse because as we both arrived at the Nurses' Station the ward went quiet, patients, relatives (it was visiting time) and other staff started to wonder what the shouting was about and they were looking at me.

The Staff Nurse shouted at me in front of the patients, their relatives and other students accusing me of something that I had supposedly done wrong. I was embarrassed, upset and extremely hurt by this accusation. Eventually, a Care Assistant admitted that she was to blame and not me. The Staff Nurse walked away without offering me an apology.

I was left to face the patients with guilty feelings for doing something that I didn't do. If I was to blame, surely the correct way to deal with the situation was to talk to me privately and not to make a public exhibition of me. Therefore, this negative experience meant that I left that placement with negative views and I feel that I never ever want to work there again. This experience had an influence on my learning whilst on the placement and although I achieved my learning outcomes thanks to other staff members, my achievements were predominantly reliant on my motivation and determination to learn and succeed.

As a mentor, what could you learn from this experience?

This is a useful case study as it identifies that although there may be potential mentorship problems, they can be converted into a positive situation. Mentorship is a satisfying experience for both mentors and students but unfortunately at times the relationship may become challenged. In contrast, operant conditioning is the feedback process that mentors use when helping students work through a systematic nursing procedure. At each stage of that procedure the mentor should give the student positive feedback so that they can progress onto the next level.

If there are negative issues, they should be dealt with in a positive manner, any misconceptions should be discussed so that the student appreciates and understands the mentor's comments and learns from them. This positive approach will help construct transferable skill development. These two approaches may offer something in contemporary healthcare. It would now be advantageous to consider the ways that a mentor could facilitate a teaching session in the practice placement.

Preparing to teach

There are just a few variables that should be considered before a teaching session or episode takes place:

1   *Who*: Who are the healthcare students? – Midwifery, nursing or allied professions.
2   *What*: What is their background? What is their level of training? What is their previous knowledge?
3   *When*: When is the teaching episode to take place?
4   *Where*: What environment or situation will be used?
5   *Why*: What is the purpose or reasoning behind the session?
6   *How*: How and in what way is the session best presented?

Now complete Mentor Activity 3.3.

MENTOR ACTIVITY 3.3

What makes a good learning experience for a healthcare student?

Answer this question and reflect on your response.

Your responses will depend on your previous experiences and approaches to practice-based teaching. Teaching in the practice placement is an entirely different experience from teaching in a classroom setting. While the practice setting could be argued to be an ideal environment for the teaching of clinical skills, the essential fusion of theoretical knowledge into practical skills can be more demanding and can call for a greater concentration and focus. What is suggested in the following is an ideal situation when taking into account the requirements of a teaching session. However, in practice, we do not always have the luxury of planning time. Some of the best learning experiences for students can be ad hoc or spontaneous. This can take particular skill, experience, expertise and the confidence of the teacher or facilitator in the practice setting. Nevertheless there are a number of things to consider when planning a teaching session.

Educational taxonomies

Consider that if we are to learn, then a change takes place. This change may be able to be measured in some way by assessment. A major figure in these changes was Benjamin Bloom (1968) who proposed that these changes would take place in certain areas and at certain levels depending upon the learning experience. He proposed that these areas be called taxonomies and they provide more detail in domains. Taxonomy is a classification. A domain is in this case an area within learning; and so Bloom's taxonomic domains refer to areas of change taking place when a student has been exposed to a learning episode. Once that learning has taken place, then it is possible to assess that change.

The taxonomic domains proposed by Bloom (1968) are:

- *The cognitive domain* refers to the knowledge, thinking and intellectual ability. The emphasis is on remembering, reasoning and creative thinking.
- *The psychomotor domain* which refers to motor skills and dexterity.
- *The affective domain* in mental health areas means mood or mental state but for educational purposes refers to attitude, emotive qualities, values and emotional attributes and bias.

In each of these areas are levels of teaching and or learning according to the level or need of the student. The levels listed are in order of increasing difficulty starting with the most basic first.

The cognitive domain

This consists of six developmental phases starting with a lower level which involves the exposure to knowledge and the upper level, being able to evaluate and make judgements (see Box 3.5).

Box 3.5   The developmental phases within the cognitive domain

1   Knowledge
2   Comprehension
3   Application
4   Analysis
5   Synthesis
6   Evaluation

---

1   *Knowledge:* This is the lowest level in this domain. It looks at the student's ability to recall facts or terms. This could be done by rote learning, e.g. the student's ability to recall the names of the twelve cranial nerves.
2   *Comprehension:* Looks at understanding and meaning, e.g. when the student is able to relate the patient's clinical features to their associated altered pathophysiology.

3 *Application*: Builds on understanding of the learned material and applies it to a particular area or need. This is demonstrated when students show the ability to relate theory taught in higher education institute to the understanding of the specific delivery of patient care in the practice placement.

4 *Analysis*: This level looks at component parts learned, breaking down the material and trying to find connections and relationships, particularly pertinent if the student is following a modular training programme.

5 *Synthesis*: This level looks at putting material together and rearranging it in a different way. Students demonstrate this when they can apply theory to patient care which is outside of the norm and is therefore individualistic rather than generalised.

6 *Evaluation*: This level looks at value judgements about the material learned. At this level of functioning a person effectively evaluates a review of the material and is likely to make suggestions for change or adaptation of material (Quinn and Hughes, 2007).

It would be helpful if mentors valued the importance of the stages within this cognitive domain and appreciated how healthcare students process the information that they are exposed to when in the practice placement. This would help in understanding the individual student's needs. Now consider the psychomotor domain (Box 3.6).

Box 3.6   The psychomotor domain

1 Perception
2 Set
3 Guided response
4 Mechanism
5 Complex overt response
6 Adaptation
7 Origination

---

1 *Perception*: The introduction to a practice task.

2 *Set*: This level looks at the process and logic of a task and the skill required.

3 *Guided response*: This looks at observing the facilitator and the discussion of the skill.

4 *Mechanism*: This looks at the learning of the logic and format of the skill.

5 *Complex overt response*: Finally, internalization takes place and the skill becomes a competency.

6 *Adaptation*: Once the skill is established, then expertise develops and a questioning takes place as to its effectiveness and other uses.

7 *Origination*: This area builds on expertise and development into other skills, other adaptations and change of use (Quinn and Hughes, 2007).

The process of healthcare delivery for nurses, midwives and allied professions involves the use of practical skills. The stages within this domain will help mentors appreciate which processes the student will go through from the stage of introducing the task to finally being able to transfer that skill to other healthcare settings. In contrast, the affective domain (Box 3.7) involves feelings.

Box 3.7   The developmental phases within the affective domain

1   Receiving
2   Responding
3   Values
4   Organization
5   Characterization by value

---

1   *Receiving*: Literally says what it means – to receive information.
2   *Responding*: Response can be complex, dependent on many things, for example, background, belief, experiences.
3   *Values*: This looks at the individual's background attitude value.
4   *Organization*: This refers to the interpretation and arrangement of that material in one's own mind.
5   *Characterization by value*: This looks at the end viewpoint based on all previous learning and offers argument, alteration and suggestion (Quinn and Hughes, 2007).

As you can see, each of these domains becomes more complex as one progresses through the levels, requiring a greater and more complex understanding not only from the student but also from the teacher or facilitator. Bloom is only one of many models for planning teaching. What mentors must remember is how these theoretical concepts can be applied to facilitating learning for healthcare students. There is no doubt that healthcare students do learn differently from each other although the basic approach remains the overarching link. Mentors have a positive, supporting role in assisting healthcare students obtain their optimum learning in the practice placements. Hence, mentors can reflect on their valued contribution and the appreciation that their student shows towards them. The process of learning can become more individualistic when the student has a learning disability. Now read Case study 3.2 for a positive student experience and the role of a supportive mentor.

CASE STUDY 3.2

A student nurse was reflecting on her practice placement experience and how supportive her mentor had been with facilitating her learning.

The student informed her mentor that she had dyslexia and although it is hard for her to learn, she would need the mentor and other staff members to tell her a few times so that she can grasp an understanding.

The mentor reassured the student that this was not a problem and she was pleased that she had been honest and open regarding her dyslexia rather than struggling throughout her placement. She confirmed that if there was anything she didn't understand, she must ask again and again in order to help her understand. This caring approach the student sincerely appreciated, resulting in a very positive learning experience for this student with subsequent acquisition of her practice proficiencies.

As a mentor, how would you deal with this situation?

Kolb (1976) developed or proposed a learning cycle looking at the following:

- *Concrete learning experiences,*
- *Reflection*: thinking the learning experience over,
- *Abstract concept*: analysis of the learning experiences,
- *Active experimentation*: concepts tested in the situation.

Kolb's learning cycle

This is a cyclical model suggesting that learning is a continuum starting as many learners do in that they require to learn something factual and useable and then to move on and to consider the learning. This moves to further reflection and an argument as to its usability, the rights and wrongs and the adaptation of the learning experience. Moving on then from this is further experimentation in other settings or ways and testing effect, and so on to setting in a concrete learning experience, and around we go again.

Teaching styles used in the practice placement

Teaching styles will be considered although the actual style should be varied according to the time, place, student and subject being taught. To adopt an authoritarian style leans more towards a didactic or dictatorship style. Here there is limited or no discussion and the teacher takes on a dominant role. This type is appropriate within higher education institutes in a lecture theatre environment but not pertinent to the practice placement.

In contrast, a Socratic style suggests a more respectful approach, asking questions and encouraging the student to answer. The teacher is not dominant but guides, supplies or leads to answers when the student does not know them (Cole, 2006). This is more appropriate for healthcare students. It will allow the mentor to identify what the student has learnt, any misconceptions or any other areas of weaknesses that need to be addressed. This approach is more relevant if the relationship between the mentor and student is going to be successful. It is a more student-led approach and correlates with adult learning philosophy of being self-directed. However, the mentor will have previously prepared the answers and these can be compared with those supplied by the student.

A heuristic style acknowledges both the teacher and students. They each possess knowledge and ignorance and both can be in a position to learn. Both have areas that the other lacks. Here more responsibility is placed on the student to find out information and the student is given respect for their involvement. This is an approach that works well in an academic classroom setting but can also be used by an effective mentor. A useful strategy for mentors is to produce learning strategies that focus on patient problems, conditions, treatments that are then converted into a scenario for discussion. Although it could be argued by mentors that this is time-consuming, it should also be viewed as a strategy that is student-led and hence appropriate for the practice placement.

A counselling style focuses on the views and feelings about the material or subject. It considers the relationship and interaction of the student and teacher. This is a sensitive approach that encourages the students to express how they felt when they were in this situation. It is emotive but can also be therapeutic if it provides a platform for the student to express their dissatisfaction with the way they were treated by their mentor or other placement staff members. Talking to students regarding their experiences (which have since been converted to the case studies used throughout this book), has helped them to rationalize how they felt and to share their success or otherwise within the mentorship relationship.

A transmission model looks at transmitting knowledge skills and attitudes to the student and Ausubel, Novak and Hanesian's (1978) model looks at assimilation, considering learning should consist of meaningful learning, discovery and overt learning or rote discovery (Quinn and Hughes, 2007). These styles offer an insight into the different styles that one has or that can be adopted, but this perhaps segregates and simplifies styles of teaching too much in that a teacher will adopt, and adapt many different approaches and styles, in order that learning can be absorbed by the student.

The teaching environment

This is probably far easier in a higher educational institute than in any practice placement, but at the same time there is arguably nothing better in learning in such an environment. Nevertheless certain proprieties need to be observed:

- The teaching/learning area needs to be organized or booked. This can be a ward or a side room or a spare room of some sort.
- The area should be conducive to learning, this needs careful consideration.
- There should be the necessary educational prompts/supports available.
- There may be basic aims and objectives but these are not well established because of the spontaneity related to some practice-based teaching sessions.
- Mentors may relate to the fundamentals of these properties but in the placement setting, the situation is different.

In practice placements, teaching or facilitation of learning is often spontaneous, related to an individual patient or student's needs, and the mentor uses their intuitive knowledge and experience to ascertain what they hope the student will achieve. The use of set objectives in the practice placement is not always appropriate for mentors, although the student's competences, outcomes or proficiencies are good indicators of what needs to be achieved and hence the focus of a teaching session. Eisner (1975) preferred to look at objectives that were more of desired outcomes that were expressive without the implication that at the end of this lesson the student would be able to do something or other. For example, Eisner's guide to objectives generally is: 'To understand, analyse, explore, explain, consider or to discuss.'

These types of objectives are more favoured by some because they look at things from a desired viewpoint, taking into account the aim of the facilitator to impart information or skills and not to assume that these will be understood immediately after the session. Some authors preferred a more exacting approach, such as Davies (1981), and looked at these descriptors as imprecise and vague. However, there has to be a point where learning has taken place and therefore should be able to be measured, but this should be considered in the assessment period. By the same token, it could be argued that it was not the intention of Bloom to make this assumption either. This would expect too much of the interaction. The intention is that after a period, of learning, revision and review over a given period, then the student may be able to perform in accordance with the desired objectives.

However, caution has to be observed here that when a healthcare student asks to be taught or shown something, it is not realistic in the clinical situation to excuse yourself for several hours while you prepare a lesson plan with aims, objectives and learning outcomes. However, this should at least help you to think logically with your presentation or learning episode. Once your learning episode has been completed, it is very useful to evaluate this episode either formally or informally. The feedback provided by the learner should hopefully be used as a guide to the effectiveness of the teaching sessions and perhaps areas or weaknesses or that need further development.

Support for students in practice

Practice dictates that some nurses are not mentors by choice. This is so for all healthcare professionals but is a compulsory inherent part of the job. When mentors are reluctant to carry out this important role, then it can put additional pressure on those who do perform their mentorship role, in accordance with their professional duties. Not everyone wants to be a mentor and this is often echoed by students as they reflect on their mentorship experiences.

What do mentors need to do to enhance their mentorship skills?

- Good leadership and a genuine encouragement of support from the staff.
- An in-built appraisal system to make mentorship part of a continuing professional development.
- Being given/allowed time to mentor within the clinical practice setting.
- Attending a yearly mentor update to maintain mentorship currency (NMC, 2008a).
- Giving feedback from student evaluations. If these have any negatives, don't be disheartened. Build on these points positively and constructively. Remember that some students will evaluate according to how they have managed to 'get their own way' or not, and some colleagues don't see the benefits of mentorship.

There can be little doubt that the personal qualities of the mentor influences the way they carry out their role and this in turn can influence the healthcare student. The *Making a Difference* document (Department of Health, 1999) places equal importance on practice as well as theory, indeed, theory can be said to only be understood when combined with practice. In this way it continues to support the importance of a mentor–student partnership. The Department of Health report states: 'Provision of practice placements is a vital part of the education process. Every practitioner shares the responsibility to support and teach the next generation of nurses/midwives.'

Throughout this chapter the focus has been on the concept of facilitation of learning in the practice placement, highlighting the aims of the NMC (2008a) Domain Two, the individual objectives as stated in both the Mentor Stage One: Nurses and Midwives and Stage Two: Registered Mentor, and with consideration to the HPC (2008). It is hoped that the primarily generic approach used throughout this chapter will help all mentors of healthcare students to facilitate the learning of their student irrespective of the specific healthcare setting. The individual theories examined may all have an influence in ensuring that mentors are aware of the individuality that they may encounter whilst mentoring their healthcare student.

Frequently asked questions

Mentors

Q. I had a first-year student nurse on his placement who wanted to arrange lots of insight visits. I was concerned that he might not achieve his placement outcomes because he seemed to be spending less and less time on the ward. How many insight visits should a student undertake?

A. The number and appropriateness of the insight visits are up to the mentor and placement staff to decide. However, the student must achieve the expected placement outcomes as a priority. If the aim of the insight visit is to enhance the student's understanding of other allied professionals' contribution to the patient's healthcare journey and they can then reflect on their learning and how it corresponds with their learning outcomes, the visit should have mutual agreement. This will contribute to facilitating the student's learning.

Q. I have a student nurse who has a weekend job and therefore will not work any weekends whilst on this placement. I am concerned because the ward is busy and there are possibly more learning opportunities to be gained by working weekends, so what should I say?

A. It is advisable for student nurses to gain a broad understanding of healthcare service delivery throughout the seven days and 24-hour day in order to facilitate their learning. At weekends the environment may be different and it is advisable for students to be aware of the differences. If in doubt, talk to the student's Personal Tutor.

Students

Q. I have completed my first placement but I am really concerned. I have produced evidence that I have achieved my placement outcomes but my mentor states that she hasn't got time to give me any feedback until my last day.

A. The NMC (2004c) states that students should produce a portfolio of evidence to verify their development and achievements. The mentor should be using continuous assessment, which means they must

(Continued)

(Continued)

give you regular feedback to inform you of your developments and achievements. Discuss this with your Personal Tutor.

Q. One of my colleagues has been working a 12-hour day because everybody else on that ward does, so can I?

A. The hours that student nurses work must correlate with those established by the higher education institute, in accordance with the NMC. In some places mentors would agree that by working along-side them for the 12-hour shift will ensure that they can directly observe you more and hopefully facilitate your learning more effectively. You need to discuss this with your mentor and Ward Leader to clarify local policy and justify that you will be able to observe continuity of care more effectively without being put at risk.

Chapter summary

This chapter has examined the importance of facilitating learning in the practice setting and the valuable contribution that the mentor can make as part of the mentorship relationship. Having completed this chapter, you have learned about:

- the individualistic variables which are pertinent to healthcare students and mentors need to understand;
- the pedagogy and andragogy approaches to teaching, their variation and how they can be applied to healthcare students;
- the importance of utilizing staff resources despite the inherent problem of time restraint;
- the significance of the learning theories: cognitivism, humanism and behaviourism and their impact in the practice placement;
- the influence of taxonomic domains in understanding the facilitation of learning of healthcare students.

Further reading

Quinn, F.M. and Hughes, S.J. (2007) *Quinn's Principles and Practice of Nurse Education.* 5th edn. London: Nelson Thornes.

This is a good all-round book looking at the theories and practice of teaching and assessing, and hence facilitation of learning.

4

Assessing healthcare students using a five-dimensional approach to assessment

David Kinnell

Nursing and Midwifery Council (2008a): Eight domains of mentorship
Domain Three: Assessment and accountability

Aim

Assess learning in order to make judgements related to the NMC standards of proficiency for entry to the register or for recording a qualification at a level above initial registration.

Outcomes

Stage 1: Nurses and Midwives

- Work to the NMC Code for nurses and midwives in maintaining own knowledge and proficiency for safe and effective practice.
- Provide feedback to others in learning situations and to those who are supporting them so that learning is effectively assessed.

Stage 2: Mentor

- Foster professional growth, personal development and accountability through support of students in practice.
- Demonstrate a breadth of understanding of assessment strategies and ability to contribute to the total assessment process as part of the teaching team.

(Continued)

(Continued)

- Provide constructive feedback to students and assist them in identifying future learning needs and actions. Manage failing students so that they may enhance their performance and capabilities for safe and effective practice or be able to understand their failure and the implications of this for their future.
- Be accountable for confirming that students have met or not met the NMC competencies in practice, and as a sign-off mentor confirm that students have met or not met the NMC standards of proficiency and are capable of safe and effective practice.

This chapter will give some suggestions and advice on meeting these requirements. Therefore, read the case studies, mentor activities and frequently asked questions and relate these to your mentorship experiences.

Introduction

There is no doubt that the mentor makes a valued contribution to the assessment of healthcare students. The mentor therefore ensures the continuity of professional practice, the maintenance of professionalism and the management of avoidable disruptions. This chapter will apply a five-dimensional model to the assessment process in an attempt to assist all mentors to approach mentorship in a logical manner. This model will consider the rationale for assessments, the components and process of assessment, before discussing the evaluation and construction of an action plan (Box 4.1).

Box 4.1   The five-dimensional assessment model for mentors

Rationale + Components + Process + Evaluation + Action Plan = Five-Dimensional Assessment Model for Mentors

---

The five-dimensional model of assessment

The assessment process can be subjective and therefore is not in reality without its inherent challenges. The five-dimensional model is a useful assessment tool that could be an aide-mémoire for mentors undertaking mentorship. The aim throughout this chapter is to ascertain if problems can be avoided and hence ensure the success of mentorship. It could be argued that the criteria of assessment should be related to the nursing and healthcare student's anticipated learning experience and be a valuable medium through which to direct the student's future learning. This could be a positive approach for both mentor and student.

This general approach to assessment will be the main focus, maintaining an interprofessional approach and be relevant to healthcare students in order to assist all mentors in practice. However, in this chapter a particular stance is directed towards nursing practice and the recommendations stipulated by the Nursing and Midwifery Council (2008a). You will need to read the aim and outcomes for Stage One: Nurses and Midwives and contrast with the Stage Two: Mentor, reflecting on how you meet the requirements in the practice area where you work. If there are any areas of concern, you could discuss these with your colleagues, educational link or use them as a focus topic at your next mentor update.

Rowntree (1997) reprinted his guidelines that provide a useful framework and constitutes the process of assessment. His framework comprises the sections: why assess, what to assess, how to assess, how to interpret and how to respond. This framework has been adapted into a five-dimensional model that is used as the basis within the mentor preparation course and for the overall structure of this chapter in order to enhance your awareness of this aspect of your role.

Now, complete Mentor Activity 4.1 before considering the significance of Case study 4.1.

MENTOR ACTIVITY 4.1

What is the rationale for an effective assessment?

Make some notes before proceeding with this chapter.

You can consider your notes as you read through the following discussion. Mentor Activity 4.1 is intended to support you and help you obtain a better understanding of assessment. However, first give some consideration to Case study 4.1.

CASE STUDY 4.1

You have a first-year student nurse who whilst assessing him presents you with some evidence that he believes verifies the achievements of his practice outcomes.

However, whilst assessing his evidence, you are not convinced that he has accomplished enough knowledge and skills in order to verify his claims. You are concerned that he is not developing the appropriate attitudes that you think he should, considering the amount of time he has been on your practice area.

You are also concerned about his apparent ineffective communication and interpersonal skills. As a mentor you want to be as helpful as possible but you also need to guide him accordingly.

What advice and guidance would you give to this junior student nurse if you were assessing his achievements, in order to maintain a positive mentorship stance?

Some areas for consideration:

1   Part of your mentor's role is to assess the ability of the student to relate theory to practice in order to ascertain their progress and development throughout their training. As a result, you should be able to identify areas that the student has failed to achieve so that these can become focus areas that they need to develop in the future. This links into the accountability component of this domain.

2   The Student Practice Placement Outcomes have been specified by the NMC (2004c), and part of the challenge of mentorship is to assist students to achieve what is expected. In a reciprocal response, the student will hopefully appreciate the efforts made and value the mentor's contribution.

3   As a mentor, you have to reiterate the importance of providing appropriate evidence in order that you can sign to verify if the evidence relates appropriately. If you are not satisfied, you must inform the student that there is insufficient evidence and hence they have not met the requirements. This will then be documented.

4   The quality of evidence and how many outcomes this student has achieved remain dependent on the mentor's professional judgement. Therefore, as a mentor you should encourage the student to reflect on the knowledge and skills that they have already developed, before highlighting areas of weakness that need further consideration. The student will hopefully see this mentorship relationship as a positive approach to helping them achieve what is expected.

5   However, the student may not always agree and hence the mentor must specify the importance of their accountability and how they are working to meet the NMC (2004c) requirements. Therefore, identifying the student's weaknesses and helping them realize these, can be a challenging yet rewarding component of mentorship assessment.

These are some suggestions to help you respond effectively in practice to Case study 4.1. However, you also need to reflect on your responses to the question in the Mentor Activity 4.1 – 'What is the rationale for an effective assessment?'

Rationale for an effective assessment

It is a statutory requirement to assess healthcare students. In particular, it is a necessity to assess student nurses during their training in order to license them as competent practitioners and subsequently protect the public (Nursing and Midwifery Council, 2008b). Furthermore, according to Rowntree (1997), only those students who are deemed competent are allowed to become registered. Therefore, according to Hinchliff (2004), it is necessary to assess the level of competence, achievement and performance related to knowledge, skills and attitudes as identified in Case study 4.1.

In contrast, Neary (2001) points out that assessments highlight weaknesses and strengths, and provides a baseline for future learning needs for the student. The opportunity for this feedback builds up confidence and guides the student to their goals (Clynes and Raftery, 2008). The standards are also maintained if learners or any other worker in the clinical area are assessed. However, there is no place for complacency, for some healthcare students assessments do produce anxiety and stress. Therefore, Nicklin and Kenworthy (2000) emphasize that assessment could detract rather than enhance learning. It can affect the effectiveness of the teacher and learner relationship, particularly if there is negative feedback which can demoralize the learner. This is a pertinent issue also highlighted by Egan (2007).

Knowles (1994) developed an approach to teaching adults known as andragogy which is a proactive approach to learning. Malcolm Knowles (1994) emphasizes the difference between the way children learn (pedagogy) and that of adults. There is an assumption that adults want to learn and this is associated with their perception of their own self-concept. It could be argued that adults value the importance of learning and have the motivation to be student-centred, and self-directed in identifying what they already know and what they need to discover. However, assessing a healthcare student can actually induce an anti-andragogical impact as the learner may not have the self-motivation, the readiness to learn, or adequate self-esteem (Cole, 2006).

Consider your responses to Mentor Activity 4.1 and contrast with Table 4.1.

TABLE 4.1   *Rationale for assessment*

- Statutory Body requirements: Introduced by the UKCC (1999) and subsequently endorsed by the Nursing and Midwifery Council (after it came into existence in 2002).

- Assessment helps to ascertain if the student is:

  Fit for purpose – can function competently in clinical practice.
  Fit for practice – can fulfil the needs of registration.
  Fit for award – have the breadth and depth of learning to be awarded a diploma or a degree (RCN, 2004: 3).

- Alternatively, from an allied professions perspective, the standards of conduct, performance and ethics apply to every registrant and prospective registrant (Health Professions Council, 2007b).

- Assess if learning has taken place and to what extent.

- Monitor the progress and development of the healthcare student.

- Identify suitability for future employment as a qualified Registered Practitioner.

- Gain feedback from patients, residents, service users, relatives, or carers regarding the healthcare student's suitability for the chosen profession, and specifically for nursing students, their selected branch: adult, child, learning disabilities or mental health. This is a valued contribution to the feedback of a student's performance but the actual final decision of achievements must be made by the mentor who has been trained to assess the knowledge, skills and development of professional attitudes.

Once the rationale for assessment has been explored, the next stage within the five-dimensional model is to examine the components of assessment in order to justify the importance of the process. Complete Mentor Activity 4.2 and try to relate to your own practice area. To fully appreciate the mentorship role, a mentor must ensure that they are aware of what is expected of them regarding assessment of students, and how the role may evolve in accordance with changes in the Student Nurse Training Programme and differing assessment strategies. Sometimes problems with mentorship arise surreptitiously, by completing Case study 4.2 the combination will encourage you to reflect on your own style of mentorship.

MENTOR ACTIVITY 4.2

What components of the healthcare student's progress do mentors assess?

Answer this question and reflect on your response.

This is intended to be a thought-provoking exercise as it encourages mentors to reflect on their particular expectations and understanding of the healthcare student's training needs. Now consider the next scenario, and reflect on your mentorship skills of how you would have dealt with the situation in Case study 4.2.

CASE STUDY 4.2

A second-year Student Nurse complains to her Personal Tutor that her mentor has not completed her Assessment of Practice Record effectively because she states that she has failed to achieve five proficiencies.

This problem had not been identified until the student's last week on placement, therefore, the mentor had provided the student with minimal assessment feedback.

The situation was made worse because the mentor had been on two weeks annual leave and apparently did not arrange for an associate or co-mentor to monitor this student's progress in their absence.

How would you deal with this situation?

This was a very difficult case study to deal with because there appeared to be faults on both sides. When asked to mediate an emotive situation like this, it needs careful planning and consideration because the mentor was blaming the student and the student nurse felt that she had been left unsupported and, therefore, was blaming the mentor.

Consider the following suggestions:

1   You need to talk to the student nurse and ascertain the facts in order to provide a plan of action.
2   It is important to highlight that it is the student's responsibility to provide evidence to correspond with achieving the NMC (2004c) proficiencies and hence their blame for failing to meet the five proficiencies.
3   You need to reiterate the role of the mentor is to verify the evidence and not produce it. However, if the student's progress had been monitored continuously, this situation could have been avoided.
4   Reiterate the range of evidence that could have been collected. It is up to the student to produce it and the mentor verifies if satisfied.
5   'Mentor on two weeks annual leave – no cover': This needs to be discussed with the mentor in order to clarify the situation. There is a need to ascertain who was the associate/co-mentor and why did they not monitor the situation.
6   The Ward Manager should have been aware that the mentor was on annual leave and arranged for alternative support.
7   There is also a need to identify why the student didn't contact the School of Nursing if she felt so vulnerable and unsupported – this situation could have been resolved more effectively.

8   It is important to remind mentors that if there is a problem with a student, they must inform the School of Nursing before the last week, so that the situation may be managed more effectively, and they can identify ways in which the student could have achieved the failed proficiencies before the last week of placement.

9   This was an emotive situation with both parties at fault and the situation could have been resolved if they had contacted the Personal Tutor or an education link from the School of Nursing for appropriate guidance.

10 How would you deal with this situation differently? What actions would you have taken? It is important to write down and record the events throughout.

11 This was an interesting situation and is not as unique as it first appears. Some students do complain that they don't see their mentor for long periods of time yet mentors are the ones to verify their achievements.

12 However, students are informed that mentorship is a two-way relationship and they must appreciate all the different demands that the mentor has to meet. If they work in collaboration with the mentor, mentorship can be a very positive and rewarding experience for all those involved.

The components of assessment

The second dimension of the five-dimensional model states that in order to be competent in their coursework, it is necessary for healthcare students to demonstrate acceptable levels of knowledge, skills and attitudes that correlate with the expectations of their specific professional body. This is supported by the achievement of practice outcomes, competencies or proficiencies that are used as an assessment tool checklist to benchmark the student's personal achievement of their development whilst caring for patients, clients or service users.

The learning achieved will be evident by observing overt behaviour, which is related to attitudes and interpersonal skills. This is demonstrated in the development and self-efficacy of the healthcare student's communication skills with patients, clients, service users and members of the inter-professional team. In contrast, practical skills and level of knowledge ideally can be assessed by questioning and direct observations. Albeit, in reality, intrapersonal skills, which include confidence, self-control, awareness of the learner's own abilities and their influence on others, may be more difficult to assess (Banning, 2005).

Hopefully within Mentor Activity 4.2 you have included some of the components identified in Box 4.2.

Box 4.2   Some of the components that mentors need to monitor in a healthcare student's progress

- Development of the healthcare student's knowledge, skills and attitudes.
- Communication and interpersonal skills.
- Attendance, punctuality, time keeping.
- Standard of patient care delivery.
- Conscientiousness, interest, motivation and willingness to learn.
- Contribution to team membership, cohesion and stability.
- Suitability for chosen profession.
- Achievement of specific competencies, outcomes or proficiencies.

Competency, according to Quinn and Hughes (2007), is associated with safety but that alone is not sufficient to make a competent practitioner. There needs to be a clear link between the facilitation of learning and the process of assessment. They advocate that the effectiveness of assessing a student is influenced by the cardinal criteria of assessment and state that every assessment must consider the following four criteria of validity, reliability, discrimination and practicality. An overview of these criteria may assist mentors in deciding the components of assessment that are pertinent to their healthcare speciality.

Cardinal criteria of assessment

Validity

Healthcare students will have their learning objectives clearly defined before they arrive on their placement. Although the assessment terminology may vary (competencies, outcomes, or proficiencies), the mentor has to assess according to the established criteria (NMC, 2004c; HPC, 2008). The term validity refers to the process whereby the assessment actually measures what it is supposed to measure. The assessment strategy is therefore designed to ensure that the appropriate components of assessment relevant to the healthcare student's training programme, are included and the validity is achievable.

The mentor's role is predominantly associated with the process of assessment in practice although they may facilitate the healthcare student's learning based on the requirements of written assignments, practice-based assessments or OSCE (Objective Structured Clinical Examination) simulation assessments, undertaken in the relevant higher education institutes.

However, the mentor must be realistic in ensuring that they are assessing what they are supposed to assess in the time constraints of the healthcare student's practice-based allocation. Therefore, which competencies, outcomes, or proficiencies the student can achieve will depend on their time allocation and the commitment shown by the healthcare student.

Reliability

Although there are clearly a number of complexities of assessment because of their subjective nature, the role of an assessment tool is to ensure that all those healthcare professionals involved in assessing students understand the criteria that are required. Therefore, irrespective of the terminology adopted, all same grade students will be assessed in the same manner using a generic specific checklist (NMC, 2004c) and not according to their popularity or personality traits. Although an idealistic stance, if an assessment is to be viewed as reliable, the assessment criteria have to be objectively utilised so that there can be a consensus of opinion: has the healthcare student achieved the stated learning outcome – yes or no?

If a reliable assessment is utilized effectively, there should not be room for discrepancy between mentors or co-mentors. Oliver and Endersby (2003) emphasized that, to be reliable, the assessment strategy must be reproducible and consistent. Therefore, although in healthcare a number of assessment strategies are used in the assessment process, they should be effectively reliable so as to produce a consensus of opinion, and valid so that they assess what is intended.

Discriminatory power

Whichever approach to assessment is adopted, the aim is to be able to identify those healthcare students who have achieved from those that have not. The ability to discriminate in a healthcare assessment is based on a professional stance and not related to negative labelling that happens in a societal manner. Throughout Mentor Preparation Training Programmes the process of assessment is explored and the need to maintain an objective, unbiased, individualistic assessment of students emphasized. Mentors are encouraged to reflect on their assessment skills in order to be able to differentiate those students who have achieved the competencies, outcomes or proficiencies from those who have not.

Healthcare students' documentation is often designed in order to map, monitor and evaluate their practice-based achievements by utilizing a tick box system. Therefore, mentors will have to discriminate in order to tick the box 'achieved' or 'not achieved' if appropriate, depending on individual performance. These cardinal criteria of assessment do assist mentors in formulating their assessment judgements providing that the last factor is also taken into consideration.

Practicality or utility

Quinn and Hughes (2007) emphasize that the assessment undertaken must be appropriate for its purpose. The assessment criteria for healthcare students have been formulated based on advice and guidance from both educationalists and practitioners. At each level of training, at the start of the training programme until the end, the assessment requirements have been agreed in accordance with the anticipated development of the student.

Therefore, mentors do need to have a clear awareness of the student's training programme, and the changes that have been implemented, in order to ensure that their knowledge is up to date. This will help validate the significance of assessment strategies used within the process and how they have been modified in order to meet changing needs and expectations of patients, clients and service users. Is the student safe?; are they putting the patient, client or service user at risk?; do they demonstrate effective communication and interpersonal skills? – these are a sample of questions that the mentor can ask whilst assessing the student's knowledge, skills and attitudes. This could be linked to local and national policies and procedures, or guidelines and recommendations (NMC, 2007b; 2008b).

The process of assessment

So far, the first two dimensions of assessment have been examined. It is important now to explore the third dimension 'the process of assessment' to help mentors understand the inter-relatedness of each within the process of mentorship.

The process of assessment focuses on a number of variables:

- Types of assessment: formative or summative.
- Approaches to assessment: continuous or episodic.
- Use of different assessment strategies.

Types of assessment

The types of assessments used for healthcare students in the practice placement by mentors can be either *formative* or *summative*, but often a combination of both approaches is utilized throughout a training programme. The formative assessment gives an evaluation of the levels of achievement, in order to identify problems and determine how to achieve the learning goals. This will hopefully occur throughout the placement duration but is documented at the intermediate or mid-placement interview that will then lead to the construction of an action plan in order to help the student's future learning by turning negative feedback into a positive way forward. The advantage of this approach is that the student will be given feedback and any areas of weakness can be discussed and developed during the rest of the placement allocation.

Formative assessments appear to be a more useful tool for increasing student motivation. They inform the student what should be learnt and how to go about it (Quinn and Hughes, 2007). It could therefore be argued that the formative assessment emphasizes the potential of the student, whereas the summative assessment focuses on the actual achievement. If used effectively, this can be viewed as one of the most important feedback processes that the mentor may undertake because it aims to help the student expand their knowledge, skills and attitudes as part of their professional development.

Summative assessments are linked to the final interview and are part of the healthcare student's ongoing assessment. However, this is one of the main criticisms by some students regarding their mentor's commitment to their continuous assessment. Some nursing students report that they received no constructive feedback until the end of their placement and hence they were not clearly aware of their effectiveness, safety or fitness for practice. Some students are told at their final interview that they have failed to achieve specifically identified competencies, outcomes or proficiencies. Although the mentor may have reasons why this happens, the delay in providing students with this negative feedback is problematic because this can present difficulties for them to remedy any stated imperfections as it is at the end of a set time and not designed for future improvement in that area (Cole, 2006). This will subsequently influence the healthcare student's perception of the effectiveness of that mentor and practice placement. Although this happens in a minority of cases, mentors do need to be aware that it could destroy the positive rapport that they have established with their healthcare student.

Approaches to assessment

The approaches to assessment are continuous or episodic. The process of continuous assessment, although it could be argued is more time-consuming for the mentor, is nevertheless more effective and the rewarding part of mentorship that enables the mentor to work smarter. By frequently discussing and reviewing the student's progress, it gives the mentor the opportunity to provide feedback to the student regarding strengths, weaknesses and areas for future development. This also allows the mentor to ascertain which competencies, outcomes or proficiencies have been achieved and those that need to be focused upon during the remainder of the student's time on placement. Providing the student with continuous or frequent constructive feedback could be viewed as one of the most effective and positive functions of mentorship as it makes the role less challenging and less demanding.

Unfortunately, at times there is a marked dichotomy between what the mentor knows that they should ideally do, and what they can actually achieve in reality because of the ever increasing demands and expectations made upon them as qualified staff. Mentors do appreciate that continuous assessment is more reliable, valid, and realistic because the assessment is being undertaken by staff known to the healthcare student with whom they have developed an effective rapport, although the time constraints can make effective assessments problematic in some placement areas.

However, discussing mentorship with healthcare students also highlights that constantly being assessed, monitored and observed can create a degree of prolonged stress, anxiety and may influence their practice achievements. In contrast, some students may be motivated by the fear of failure and appreciate the continuous feedback from their mentors. This allows a realistic time framework if the student is aware that on a regular specified date and time their mentor will discuss, sign and verify their weekly achievements.

Continuous assessment gives mentors the opportunity to praise the student and, if it is necessary, to give them negative feedback, this can be undertaken in a positive manner from which the individual can develop (Duffy and Hardicre, 2007a). Any areas of concerns or competencies, outcomes or proficiencies that it is anticipated will not be achieved can be discussed with the student so that they develop a positive action plan to counteract those deficiencies.

Unfortunately, this is an idealistic stance and not always the approach adopted by mentors, possibly because of the sensitivity of telling the healthcare student that they are not achieving what they should or they are not at the expected standard. Some mentors feel uncomfortable about giving negative feedback but as part of mentor preparation, they are encouraged to use other colleagues or educational staff to manage this situation and convert this into a positive end product. However, some mentors adopt an episodic approach to their assessment of healthcare students. An episodic approach has a number of negative connotations attached as the student is assessed at a predetermined time and place, and not as part of an ongoing developmental programme. The essence of this approach is unrealistic because the student can prepare for the assessment rather than it being a spontaneous exploration of practice achievements. The main inherent problem associated with this approach lies with its timing.

Students report that they were given very little feedback throughout their placement experience and there were no indications that they were not actually up to standard. The ideology of mentorship then becomes problematic if the student does not receive negative feedback until the last week, or worse, the last day of placement. If this episodic approach is followed, what opportunity has the student been allowed to achieve what their mentor has identified as being an area of failure? Fortunately, this is not the approach adopted by effective mentors as they tend to discuss their students progress throughout the placement allocation.

Now read Case study 4.3 to share the experience that a student nurse had on placement which involved mentors wanting to mentor but the time constraints becoming problematic.

CASE STUDY 4.3

A second-year student nurse discussed his concerns regarding his current placement. Throughout his training so far, he had worked with very supportive mentors who had helped to facilitate his learning and encouraged his practice-based achievements.

His concern was that now he had two mentors but neither seemed to be interested in him or his achievements, to the extent he felt like a 'burden'. This was a new experience and one that caused him to feel anxious, uncomfortable, upset and distressed to the extent that he didn't want to go to work.

This community-based placement meant that he was left in an office and told to do some work on his assignment, when he really wanted to go with the mentors and visit clients that they were working with. Otherwise, how was he to learn?

Although there may be times when it is not appropriate to visit a client in their own home because of the sensitivity, confidentiality or the client's choice, this was not the case for this student. On several occasions, one mentor went directly to hold a clinic in a different location without even telling the student. Again, he was left unsupported in a placement not knowing what to do and unaware of how he was being assessed.

He was concerned with the assessment of his progress. Previous mentors had provided him with frequent feedback about his communication and inter-personal skills, identifying any areas of weaknesses in his knowledge, skills or attitudes. This had given him a focus to help him develop. Unfortunately, the lack of constructive feedback meant that he wasn't sure how his mentors were assessing him so he discussed his concerns with a lecturer from the School of Nursing.

The student returned to placement and managed to discuss his concerns and feelings with one of his mentors who acknowledged the importance of his anxiety. An action plan was devised that covered the next few weeks and ensured that the student was involved more effectively. He worked on producing a range of evidence that verified his achievements so that his mentors could assess his development and assessment of his proficiencies.

The two mentors were busy and for various reasons found that having a student to mentor was extra to the overstretched work load. Although this relates to the dichotomy between wanting to mentor a student and the reality of actually having to mentor with its inherent responsibility, it is not a situation unique to this case study. This is a discussion topic area that is often identified at face-to-face mentor update sessions. This student discussed his concerns and consequently the situation was resolved.

As a mentor involved in a similar situation, how would you deal with this more effectively?

This is an interesting case study that highlights that some mentors expect their students to be involved in more self-directed study than others but whichever assessment strategy is adopted, the mentor must ensure that the student understands the process. The use of different assessment strategies infers that individuality of the healthcare student is paramount in undertaking an effective unbiased assessment. Hinchliff (2009) warns that it is important not to prejudge the needs and abilities of students, based on what someone else has said prior to their arrival on placement. Unfortunately, if a student has had a negative experience on one placement, that information may arrive at their next area before they do. If staff respond to this information it may escalate into negative labelling and a negative self-fulfilling prophecy that may then overshadow the student's progress, and, hence, the mentorship experience will be extremely biased. In order to avoid this assessment anomaly, mentors are encouraged to utilize criterion-referencing and avoid the bias approach of norm-referencing.

Evaluation of learning

The fourth dimension of the five-dimensional approach to assessment is the evaluation of learning. Healthcare students arrive in the practice setting with specific assessment criteria to achieve. Irrespective of assessment terminology (competencies, outcomes or proficiencies, NMC, 2004b; HPC, 2004; 2007c; 2007d; 2007e; 2007f), students will have a specific checklist guiding them as to what they need to achieve and under the guidance of their mentor, these will be attained.

The principle of criterion-referencing requires students to provide evidence that they have achieved the specified criteria according to those stated by the specific guiding professional body. This should be an objective and individualistic assessment of the healthcare student's achievements. In marked contrast, some mentors use norm-referencing which is problematic because of its subjectivity and the way that it does not highlight individual student's success and development. The mentor will compare how 'good' one healthcare student is with another, instead of emphasizing individual success and progress. This may lead to a marked differentiation in mentor expectations and variation in acceptable level of standards of care. Mentorship should be a positive experience with both the mentee and the mentor aware of each other's expectations.

Bradshaw (1998) emphasizes that nursing involves the integration of cognitive (understanding), affective (emotional) and psychomotor (practical) elements and that a good assessment should ascertain achievement in all these aspects. However, she states: 'This issue of nursing competency rests in the greater issue of what constitutes a competent nurse and how she is prepared for the professional role' (1998: 103).

Although specific to nursing, this could also be extrapolated to the other specialities within the interprofessional team. Assessment in healthcare examines the rationale for assessment, the components and associated process. However, the next two sections will explore the evaluation of assessment and the construction of a resultant action plan. Mentorship is an important, interesting and challenging component of a qualified Registered Practitioner's role, at times it is also somewhat frustrating particularly if the healthcare student does not appear to be achieving the expected practice-based requirements. Therefore the mentor must appreciate and value that the assessment must remain objective and not subjective.

The effective evaluation of a healthcare student's behaviour may be influenced by the impact of the 'Three Hs' – the horn, halo and Hawthorne effects. Depending on the rapport and professional relationship between the mentor and healthcare student, there is the potentiality that the evaluation of learning is thwarted by the personality of the student. If a mentor is working with a student who is introverted, quiet, and tends to spend more time in direct care delivery rather than socializing with the team, their achievements may be 'under-rated' in accordance with the 'horn' effect. This is difficult to objectively manage and may lead to problems with verifying the individual's development. In contrast, the 'halo' effect is the opposite and occurs when the mentor 'over-rates' the student because they are more outgoing, extroverted, and sociable. This subjective misdemeanour can be problematic particularly if colleagues don't agree because they are truly on the perimeter looking inwards (Rowntree, 1997; Quinn and Hughes, 2007).

It could be argued that the third 'H' is as difficult as the first two for mentors to manage. In healthcare, it can be complex for mentors to truly evaluate the student's progress because of the 'Hawthorne' effect. This is the process by which a healthcare student deliberately demonstrates manipulative behaviour whenever they are being directly observed by their verifying mentor. The student can 'put on a performance' because they are aware that they are being observed and want to impress their mentor.

However, a controversy arises when the student is not working with that verifying mentor because they may not work to the same standard or display the same extent of enthusiasm when working with the rest of the team. Therefore, what other team members observe may not be the same as their verifying mentor – this controversy can lead to conflict if not managed in a professional manner. The mentor must ensure that the student realizes that mentorship is a team effort and individual staff members do comment on the student's behaviour, and that those comments are a valuable contribution in order to assess a collective overview of their progress and development.

In summary, the mentor's evaluation of assessment may be influenced by the following variables:

- feedback from patients, clients or service user;
- feedback from relatives or carers;
- feedback from colleagues and members of the interprofessional team;
- the extent to which the mentor is objective rather than subjective;
- the student's achievement of competencies, outcomes or proficiencies;
- mentor's own standards, quality of care delivery and adherence to benchmarking;
- assessment bias – horn, halo or Hawthorne effect.

Feedback and action plan

The final stage of the 'five-dimensional model of assessment' relates to the process of giving and receiving feedback in order to produce a supportive action plan. The mentor will be providing feedback to student using a continuous assessment process so that if there are any weaknesses or areas for future development, the student will have the opportunity to be able to discuss these.

One of the most satisfying, rewarding and self-fulfilling aspects of the mentor's role is being able to provide positive, and constructive feedback to their student (Clynes and Raftery, 2008). This will cement the mentor and healthcare student's relationship, and is seen as a positive experience for both involved. However, just as important and more difficult to execute is providing the student with negative feedback. However, if planned and discussed effectively, this negative encounter can be converted into a positive and viable experience for the student by encouraging them to document in an action plan.

The response to assessment is in the format of a written report, verbal feedback such as discussion and questioning, and the interpretation of indicative non-verbal behaviour including body language, posture, facial expression and eye contact. It is important to find an area or quiet room that will allow discussion without any interference or interruptions.

The mentor should be sensitive to the needs and feelings of the student in order to enhance their self-esteem. It is more productive to be calm and objective in order to be helpful to the student, rather than angry and defensive. In order to undertake a negative feedback, it is a paramount requirement that there is sufficient time allocated for delivery of the results, assimilation by the student and then discussion of the consequences by constructing a realistic action plan. It is therefore important that the mentor is clear and concise when giving the feedback, subsequently encouraging the student to comment and explain any issues or concerns generated. This will help the student to learn from the experiences.

Developing an action plan will encourage the student to review the mentor's feedback as constructive and guiding the way forward. The actual format is individualistic but the healthcare student does need to be aware of the importance of using an action plan in order to help them develop any areas identified as a weakness or not achieved. An action plan can then be taken to the next placement and start the mentorship process there by highlighting the areas that need to be the main focus for the next mentor to help the student with their development.

For some students, the action plan could comprise a SWOT analysis, but other models are available. If this is used as an educational tool, the student will be able to identify their:

Strengths
Weaknesses
Opportunity
Threats

A SWOT analysis will generate the opportunity for self-assessment, encouraging the healthcare student to identify both their positive and negative attributes. The mentor will therefore be able to guide the student to reflect on their progress and development, highlighting areas that need to be further developed on their next placement. The value of an action plan is that the student should construct the content themselves within the four strands of a SWOT analysis.

The mentor can encourage the student to reflect on their initial expectations that they brought to the placement and to what extent these have been achieved. Providing the student with positive feedback on their strengths establishes that progress has been made. However, some students and mentors have difficulty discussing the weaknesses as this can be seen as a negative and destructive interaction. Therefore, the mentor must be able to elaborate the importance of this self-awareness so that the evaluation can be converted into a constructive, positive action plan.

The student will be encouraged to ascertain their own progress, identify the competencies, outcomes or proficiencies achieved and those that remain outstanding. The mentor must make every effort to help the student conceptualize how the identified weaknesses can become positive achievements. It is important that this is documented in an action plan so that future developments can be monitored.

The student must also be encouraged to review the opportunities that are available and how these could be used in order to help them achieve their placement assessment criteria. In most healthcare settings, mentors construct an itinerary or list of insights visits which is the opportunity to visit other related healthcare settings that are linked to that specific placement. Spending some time with the other allied professions will hopefully assist the student to gain an appreciation of their individual role within the patient's healthcare journey. The student could use the opportunity to help them develop the areas of weaknesses identified in their action plan.

However, they must also be aware that these visits must be arranged and negotiated under the guidance of their mentor or the experience may be viewed as a threat. The timing, aims and objectives of any insight visits must be established so that the experience can be linked to the student's development and achievement of competency, outcome or proficiency. Some students may wish to undertake an insight visit that is not clearly related to their present practice placements. The mentor may discourage this because the anticipated aim and learning outcomes may be blurred. The student may see this as a threat but need to remember that their mentor is the qualified professional and they may not be able to relate the experience to the training programme.

Iles and Sutherland (2001) explore the concept and experiences of undertaking a SWOT analysis both in healthcare and industry. From the student's perspective, once they have completed their self-evaluation, they can then be encouraged to design the goals that will ultimately stimulate the construction of their action plan. An action plan helps to monitor the progress and development achieved. Although the visual format may vary, the ideology could be useful to the healthcare student as part of their continued personal and professional development.

Mentors need to provide students with feedback in an appropriate, constructive and supportive manner so that they can learn from that experience (see Box 4.3).

> **Box 4.3   Providing healthcare students with feedback**
>
> - Feedback must be constructive and not destructive.
> - Negative feedback must be given in a positive way.
> - The feedback must highlight strengths as well as weaknesses.
> - It must emphasize areas for development and improvement.
> - Praise must be given accordingly depending on achievements.

Complexities of assessment

The five-dimensional model of assessment can be viewed as a useful and influential framework that is thought-provoking but also practical in its application. However, although the individual five dimensions are inter-related, they are not without their inherent complexities because of the nature of human existence. The fascination of mentorship is indicative in its feedback from both mentors and healthcare students. Discussing experience with both groups, it is apparent that mentorship becomes less effective for a number of reasons.

From personal experiences, working with both groups over a number of years, it has become evident that no matter what contribution is made by either member in the mentorship partnership, a number of problems may arise that could threaten the end product. The following is a list of 'mentorship complexities' that need to be discussed and explored in order to understand why mentorship can become so controversial and why mentors need to maintain a positive stance towards their mentorship role.

Mentor complexities include:

- Personality clash between mentor and student.
- Variation in expectations from both parties.
- Mentors may experience difficulty dealing with subjectivity and trying to maintain an objective stance.
- Assessing individuality in healthcare students: need to consider the student's learning style, learning needs, learning disability such as dyslexia, etc.
- Personality traits of both mentor and student.
- Time constraints: on a busy placement, effectively assessing student's knowledge, skills and attitudes can be demanding especially if the student is constructing a student portfolio of evidence to meet their placement competencies, outcomes or proficiencies.
- The effectiveness of the environment may have an impact on the success of assessing a healthcare student:
- Physical environment = what resources and equipment are available in practice to assess the development of the student's skills – may be limited.

- Social environment = assessing a student in a hospital or community setting may have individual variables – does the student feel safe and secure?
- Psychological environment = the success of developing the student's intra-personal covert variables, their thoughts, feelings and aspirations may influence the overt behaviour displayed.

If these issues do cause the mentor concern, they must discuss with the student and educational link so that the ideology of mentorship remains a rewarding and positive facet of their professional role.

Frequently asked questions

Mentors

Q. What do I do if my student doesn't provide me with sufficient evidence for me to assess and sign them off?

A. The evidence to verify achievement is the student's own responsibility and should be provided for the mentor to assess. If they don't provide you with sufficient evidence they must be informed, and if they don't respond, it will be documented that they have failed the outcome/proficiency due to insufficient evidence.

Q. Whilst assessing one piece of evidence, how many outcomes or proficiencies can a student achieve?

A. The quality of the piece of evidence and not the quantity will justify what has been achieved. If you are unsure, discuss with a mentor colleague or educational link.

Students

Q. My mentor complains about the jargon in the Assessment of Practice Record and doesn't understand what it means. What can I do?

A. The jargon quoted in the Assessment of Practice Record is provided by the NMC (2004c) and hence, is a statutory requirement. If the mentor needs to discuss this, they must contact their educational link or the lecturer who delivers the Mentor Training Programme. The mentor can discuss this at their face-to-face mentor update.

Q. My mentor is always complaining about the amount of time it takes to read my practice evidence of achievement and therefore says that she

(Continued)

(Continued)

will only look through the evidence when she has time. In six weeks, we have only discussed this once. What can I do to make it easier for her?

A. The mentor should be using continuous assessment and therefore should be reviewing and verifying your evidence on a regular basis. This is mentorship.

This is a sample of a number of questions generated by mentors at mentor update sessions and student nurses at their reflection on practice sessions. Throughout this chapter, these have been addressed in an attempt to help the process of mentorship be more effective for you and your students.

Chapter summary

The overall content of this chapter has examined the process of assessment using a five-dimensional model and has encouraged you to reflect on your style of mentorship. Having completed this chapter you have learned about:

- the rationale for an effective assessment and its importance for all nursing and healthcare students, ensuring safety for those that they care for as well as meeting statutory requirements;
- the components of assessment focus on acquiring knowledge, skills and attitudes that students must develop throughout their specific training programme. The mentor must contribute to this development by offering guidance and support;
- the assessment process and how it involves the types of approaches to assessment as well as using different assessment strategies;
- the mentor's evaluation of assessment can be influenced by a number of variables that will help them to decide if the student is competent and therefore safe for practice;
- constructive feedback will allow the student to know their level of achievement and if there are any areas for further development that need to be incorporated into an action plan in preparation for their next placement.

Further reading

Downie, C.M. and Basford, P. (eds) (2003) *Teaching and Assessing in Clinical Practice: A Reader.* London: Greenwich University Press.

This book is a compilation of a number of chapters produced by a selection of authors including Oliver and Endersby, Rowntree, Girot and Milligan. Collectively, the content explores a number of issues associated with the process of assessment and its inherent complexities. Mentors should find this book useful in extending their awareness and understanding of this vital role within the remit of mentorship.

5

Evaluating the effectiveness of mentorship

David Kinnell

Nursing and Midwifery Council (2008a): Eight domains of mentorship
Domain Four: Evaluation of learning

Aim

Determine strategies for evaluating learning in practice and academic settings to ensure that the NMC standards of proficiency for registration or recording a qualification at a level above initial registration have been met.

Outcomes

Stage 1: Nurses and Midwives

- Contribute information related to those learning in practice, and about the nature of learning experiences, to enable those supporting students to make judgements on the quality of the learning environment.

Stage 2: Mentor

- Contribute to evaluation of student learning and assessment experiences, proposing aspects for change resulting from such evaluation.
- Participate in self- and peer-evaluation to facilitate personal development and contribute to the development of others.

This chapter will give you some suggestions and advice on meeting these requirements. Therefore, read the case studies, mentor activities and frequently asked questions and relate these to your mentorship experiences of gaining feedback from students' evaluation of placement.

Introduction

The process of evaluation is regarded as an essential component within the mechanism of quality assurance. Mentors and students are exposed to a variety of evaluation approaches from patient care to facilitation of learning. Students are asked to reflect on their practice experience and complete a questionnaire that reflects on the overall process of mentorship. However, some of the resultant comments may be viewed with some scepticism because of evaluation bias. Mentors can be involved in the process of educational audit which allows the placement staff to complete a questionnaire, discuss its content during an educational audit visit by a university staff member, so that any areas of concern can be expressed and any improvements for the future identified.

Box 5.1 presents an example of the process of evaluation. This can be viewed as one of many approaches of examining the stages involved in the evaluation process and will therefore form the structural framework throughout this chapter.

Box 5.1   The process of evaluation

Feedback → Review Comments → Discuss → Implement Change

Process of evaluation: feedback of practice learning

The process of evaluation is an integral dimension of all aspects of healthcare, including mentorship. Student nurses are introduced to evaluation as part of the 'nursing process', whereby they are involved in the assessing, planning, implementing, and evaluating of a patient's nursing problem and the effectiveness of the resultant plan of care. They are encouraged to develop their evaluative skills and apply them when in the practice placement. Also, they can appreciate the importance and significance of evaluation particularly if an aspect of care needs to be amended, in order to correspond to the change in the patient's condition. Therefore, they can contribute in a positive manner to the patient's healthcare journey.

However, students are also exposed to a number of other evaluations that they do not always appreciate. In the academic environment students are asked to complete a number of different types of evaluation (see Box 5.2).

Box 5.2   Types of student evaluations

- Student Evaluation of Placement
- Student Evaluation of Teaching – a specific session
- Student Evaluation of the Teaching – general
- Student Evaluation of a Module
- Student Evaluation of the Common Foundation Programme
- Student Evaluation of overall Training Programme

Although the types of student evaluation may vary according to the individual higher institutions, gaining feedback from students regarding an individual teacher's teaching strategy, either specific or collectively, could be viewed as a valuable quality assurance audit mechanism. The individual teacher receives the group's overall feedback and they are then encouraged to respond to any areas of improving the concerns identified. This is contrasted with the student's evaluation of a specific module, and how effectively the teacher has ensured that the module aims, objectives and associated assessment, were achieved. The students are asked to complete an evaluation of the Common Foundation Programme and also, one at the end of their specific branch programme. From an academic perspective all these sources of student evaluations are valued and respected, however, some of the negative comments are viewed objectively in contrast with the collective whole. Depending on the individual higher education institution the actual evaluation questionnaire and frequency of gaining student evaluation may differ. However, from both the academic and the mentors' viewpoint, the student's evaluation of placement is an important feedback process.

Student evaluation of placement

At the end of each practice placement each student is asked to complete an evaluation of that placement by providing either a paper copy or complete an electronic feedback questionnaire. They are asked to reflect on their practice placement and comment on the experience that they have gained based on four dimensions:

- the mentorship process;
- the available learning resources;
- their mentor;
- the quality of the practice placement.

The actual evaluation form content may vary but these four categories are one example. The subsequent evaluation data gained from the feedback are useful in order to assist the practice placement staff, and particularly the mentor, gain an awareness of the quality of experience gained by the student. However, the actual usefulness and effectiveness of the feedback in order to improve the placement for future students are debatable and will depend on how constructive the student has been.

The following is an example of evaluation feedback though each higher education institute will have their own specific questionnaire tool (see Box 5.3). Now complete Mentor Activity 5.1 by reflecting on your own experience.

Box 5.3   Mentorship process audit questionnaire

1   I received an introductory pack to the placement
2   I undertook orientation/induction programmes in accordance with the assessment documentation:

   (a)   Orientation 1 – during the first day,
   (b)   Orientation 2 – during the first week.

3   My preliminary interview facilitated:

   (a)   The identification of my learning needs
   (b)   The identification of learning opportunities
   (c)   The formulation of an action plan.

4   My intermediate interview facilitated discussion about my progress on the placement.
5   My final interview facilitated an effective evaluation of my achievement on this placement.
6   My final interview facilitated action planning for the future.

MENTOR ACTIVITY 5.1

What is the process of gaining evaluations of practice experience from healthcare students in your practice placement?

Answer this question before continuing so that you are aware of your local evaluation.

The feedback from mentors indicates that there are various ways in which practice placement staff respond to these students' evaluations of their experiences in a healthcare setting. In some areas there is a serious commitment to examining the feedback, identifying both the positive and negative aspects of the evaluation comments. The positive comments need to be disseminated to all the team in order that they realize that their contributions to mentorship are valued and have contributed towards that student's professional development.

Unfortunately, negative evaluation may be received as a form of unjustifiable criticism because of evaluation bias, particularly if used as a retaliation mechanism. However, this is not always the response from placement staff as these comments are examined, explored more objectively and if possible, an action plan will be constructed in order to prevent further negative feedback. You can consider your notes from Mentor Activity 5.1 as you read through the chapter. However, first give some consideration to Case study 5.1.

CASE STUDY 5.1

A third-year student nurse, in her final semester, reflected on the experience of mentorship that she had had for the last two and half years with a negative overview. She was contributing as part of a classroom discussion that was focusing on the reality and quality of mentorship.

This student was annoyed that on two branch-related placements she was made to feel like she was a *'burden'* to the mentors and that they did not really want to be a mentor. She was upset that mentors could treat students in such an unfriendly manner and to make someone feel the way that they had made her feel. It had been difficult to achieve her proficiencies on these two placements because the mentors said that they really had not the time to verify the evidence in her Student Portfolio until her last week of placement.

After the way she was treated, she was then expected to give positive feedback in her evaluation of the two placements. The mentors both stated that they had previously received good placement evaluations and that they were hoping to continue this trend. They did not like students who were negative about their mentorship experience.

The student felt that she had to give 'positive' face-to-face evaluation to the mentors because she wanted them to sign to verify the placement proficiencies. However, the student found that she was able to honestly reflect on her feelings as part of the on-line student evaluation of placement.

During the classroom discussion, this was *not* a unique or rare situation.

Consider your own mentorship experiences, are there any occasions that you think could have been viewed as a negative experience for the student – what could you do to ensure that this would not be repeated?

Exploring a negative case study in a constructive manner is a positive learning experience which the mentor can benefit from for their future professional and mentorship development.

The Royal College of Nursing (2004) provides some useful points to consider when evaluating the practice placement, these are useful for both the student and their mentor. Mentors should be aware that students will be encouraged to consider the following:

- As every placement will be different, so each evaluation is individual.
- Learn to evaluate all your practice placement experiences – good and not so good.
- Welcome feedback and learn from it.
- Ask your mentor how you have done – did your nursing care meet professional standards and safety?
- Identify how you think you have done.
- Compare your perceptions.
- Look at setbacks as opportunities for growth.
- Look for positive situations as you progress through the programme.
- Listen and connect with others.
- Remember that learning is a process, not an event.
- Ask yourself: what have I learnt? What do I need to learn more about?
- Be honest.
- Plan for your next placement.

This is a really effective checklist from the RCN (ibid.: 9) that helps to objectively consolidate the importance of evaluating practice placement experience as a positive learning experience. Kerridge (2008) reviews the experience gained by student nurses on placement within a nursing home. She specifies the significance and ever increasing demand that students place on the practice staff. Relating to Hutchings et al. (2005), Kerridge (2008) emphasizes that practice staff, including mentors, have to balance these increasing demands made on them by both patients and healthcare students. The process of evaluation is a vehicle for reality, helping to identify what it is that students perceive mentorship is, what they hope it will help them achieve and how it fails to meet their expectations and educational needs.

Clynes and Raftery (2008) explore the importance of feedback and how this is an important contribution to students evaluating their practice placement experience. Students frequently complain that mentors do not provide them with constructive feedback which they see as an essential part of the evaluation of their progress, and how they are developing their professional knowledge, skills and attitudes. Feedback is important for students in order to help them identify areas of strengths, weaknesses and further development that they need to focus on in order to achieve their outcomes or proficiencies throughout their practice placement. The process of feedback involves a number of stages (see Box 5.4).

Box 5.4   Process of feedback

- What is feedback?
- The benefits of feedback for student and supervisor.
- Student experiences of feedback.
- Barriers to giving and receiving feedback.
- The feedback process.
- Understanding students' responses to feedback.

(Clynes and Raftery, 2008).

This checklist from Clynes and Raftery (2008) could be adopted as a useful evaluation tool that will explore the healthcare student's practice placement experience from different dimensions. They state: 'Feedback on clinical performance is essential for effective student learning in clinical practice. However, students report variable experiences of receiving feedback while on practice placements', (ibid.: 40a). The effectiveness of how mentors provide students with feedback could well influence their evaluation of that placement, and dominate the stance they take on constructive objectivity or destructive subjectivity.

Healthcare students expect their mentors to evaluate the commitment that they have shown to their training as displayed in their overall behaviour. The feedback process is the vehicle for transmitting that assessment evaluation. Clynes and Raftery (ibid.: 406) state: 'Terms used to describe feedback may be categorized into two broad groups: constructive/corrective/negative and reinforcing/positive.' Feedback that mentors give to healthcare students should be based on direct observations rather than on the biased feedback from other staff members. However, the Hawthorne effect must not be disregarded, because some students may put on a performance to impress their mentor so colleagues' objective feedback must be viewed with the sincerity that it is intended to be acknowledged with.

Some students may criticize the quality and infrequency with which they are given feedback about their development and progress, and hence their negative evaluative comments may be justified. The need for regular, constructive and objective feedback has been expressed by students as a valuable component within the mentorship relationship. Welch (1999) explores the importance of evaluation in the problem-solving process related to management strategies. If a mentor has a problem with a student, they need to assess the extent of the problem, plan how they will deal with that problem, implement the action plan and evaluate its effectiveness. The process of evaluation can be viewed as a reciprocal process whereby the student and mentor both appreciate each other's contribution in the mentorship partnership.

Now complete Mentor Activity 5.2 and as you do, try to appreciate why the evaluation process is so important to your own practice area.

MENTOR ACTIVITY 5.2

What happens to the evaluations that your placement receives from healthcare students?

Identify your practice placement feedback process before proceeding with this section.

Consider the following:

- How do students evaluate your practice placement learning?
- Which evaluation tool is utilized?
- When the evaluation feedback is obtained, what happens to the student's comments?
- How are the students' comments disseminated to the mentorship team and other staff members?
- To what extent are the student's comments valued?
- How would change be initiated in response to the student's constructive feedback?

This should be an interesting activity that encourages you to be reflective and ensure that you gain an awareness of your practice placement procedure of responding to student's evaluations and reviewing the effectiveness of work-based learning.

Work-based learning has been explored by Spouse (2001), and more recently Kerridge (2008). Spouse (2001: 12) states: 'For many people work reflects their identity, often providing a meaning to their life that is reflected in social interactions.' However, she also emphasizes that within the work culture the status of the healthcare student is threatened as they work within a team of qualified professionals who are focused on their career having chosen to specialize in that specific healthcare setting. Spouse advocates that within a culture of work-based learning, the mentor and practice placement staff should want to help the student gain the most from the learning opportunities available. The mentor needs to help the student realize that although the patients' condition, aetiology, presenting clinical features, and management may be similar, the individuality of the person can make their healthcare journey unique.

The importance of work-based learning can be viewed as the process of bringing together of self-knowledge, expertise in the workplace, and formal knowledge, thereby relating theory to practice. It is therefore important for mentors to ensure that this approach is developed in healthcare students, encouraging them to reflect on their practice experience, and how it relates to the theoretical concepts discussed in the academic environment. Kerridge (2008) emphasizes that providing effective practice placements for students that will help them develop their professional knowledge, skills and attitudes remains a problematic attainment. This is often identified in the students' evaluations.

However, Wilkinson (1999) and Watson and Harris (2000) do highlight that care must be exercised when supporting and assessing students in the practice placement. Wilkinson (1999) particularly focuses on the validity and reliability of undertaking an assessment of a student's developmental abilities highlighting that it must be viewed as it is intended to be.

Now consider Case study 5.2, reflect on your mentorship skills, and identify what you can learn from this situation. This is an important case study because potentially it could have been received as a negative feedback but in reality, the mentors decided to adopt a positive and proactive stance which did and continues to benefit future students to that practice placement. This was a positive learning experience for the mentors involved, allowing them to work together and share their ideas in an attempt to produce a worthwhile team response.

CASE STUDY 5.2

At a recent mentor update discussion, a mentor reflected on the last few groups of students' evaluation of that practice placement. The comments were varied and generally constructive.

Their experiences of mentorship had been positive as they found the team helpful, reliable and worked well together to ensure that the students' learning experiences were as interesting and varied as possible.

(Continued)

(Continued)

However, there had been comments regarding the lack of resources that they could access and what was available needed to be updated and maintained to reflect current research findings. Initially receiving negative feedback is a little upsetting but these mentors in this practice placement had responded positively to those student evaluations.

As a result, the mentors decided to work together to review the existing educational resources that were accessible and they allocated a time frame in which to improve what was available. The team were very motivated, committed and revitalized their own interests in specific areas of their nursing speciality and improved their designated learning area with more appropriate and updated resources.

These mentors found the constructive evaluation useful and responded to the students' comments.

How could you respond to your students' evaluations?

How well do you accept negative criticism and do you dismiss the comments or convert them into a positive way forward? Mentorship is an important part of the student's practice placement experience, they are the 'consumers', their comments can be very thought–provoking, but working in partnership is useful.

Review students' evaluation comments

Students are encouraged to reflect on the whole placement experience and evaluate what was good, what areas caused them concern and state how the placement could be improved for future students. The comments are valued and reviewed in the context in which they were completed. Mentors should be able to ascertain for themselves how well the experience went for their student, however, there may be a need to consider evaluation bias. Sometimes, despite planning the experience in order to facilitate and enhance the student's learning as effectively as possible, the healthcare student may not always appreciate the significance of the motivation and commitment that has been involved. Mentors are therefore concerned when they read negative evaluations and try to understand why students evaluate their placement the way that they do.

Why do students evaluate the way that they do?

The process of evaluation is significant both for practice placements and the academic programme co–ordinators in order to monitor the student's progress. However, the student's comments may display aspects of evaluation bias because of intra- and/or inter-personal factors.

Intra-personal factors (internal – within the person):

- Personality clash between them, the mentor or another staff member.
- The student may have felt that they were treated differently, unfairly or discriminated against in some way, particularly if there were more than one student on that placement.
- There may be some perceptual distortion whereby the mentor does not see how ineffective the placement had been from the student's perspective.
- The personality of the student may dominate their evaluative feedback despite the mentor's conscientious efforts.
- Whatever is happening in the student's social world may influence their emotions and hence the quality of their quantitative or qualitative evaluation.
- The student's negative attitude may be influenced by the fact that they are on a placement, branch or non-branch that they did not want to work on.
- They may want to humiliate the mentor for personal reasons and hope that their negative evaluation may hurt the mentor.

Inter-personal factors (external – between two or more people):

- The mentor is exercising a procedural nomothetic approach (all students want the same experience) rather than appreciating the need for an idiographic, individualistic experience that relates to the student's previous achievements and their current specific learning outcomes that they wanted to accomplish.
- The ineffectiveness of the mentor's communication and interpersonal skills may have influenced the negative way that they treated the student.
- Students do not like to be told they lack motivation, enthusiasm or interest, so by giving negative feedback about the mentor may be seen as a retaliation mechanism.
- If the mentor has embarrassed the student in front of other students, staff members or patients, giving negative evaluation may be a way of achieving psychological closure.

Mentors therefore need to examine the students' evaluation of placement in an objective manner, identify any areas of concern and discuss with colleagues how these can be converted into a positive action plan for potential future development and change. The inevitable question that students are asked is why they didn't inform their mentor whilst on placement that there were areas of concern. For some students, the fear that their mentor will not sign to verify their achievements or the trouble that they may cause them with the academic staff, is a serious threat whilst they are on placement. Therefore, when they return to the safe haven of the academic environment, then they will evaluate how they truly felt when in the practice placement providing the subsequent negative evaluative comments.

Alternatively, the case studies throughout this book are all genuine and were shared by the students involved because they wanted somebody to listen to their fears, concerns and phenomenological accounts of mentorship. Therefore, student evaluations can also be viewed as areas of concern particularly when they identify aspects of mentorship that do not correspond to the NMC's (2008a) recommendations. These evaluations are important because they identify mentors who need to attend a mentor update or for their academic representative to discuss with them the anomaly in their practice and management of the healthcare student. Students must be reassured that their evaluations will be examined from an objective stance in order to identify areas of concerns. Conversely, some students do print inappropriate, hurtful and almost damaging comments that need to be treated with a professional sensitivity. The RCN (2004: 16) presents a useful checklist of factors for students to consider on completion of their placement and provide a 'yes' or 'no' response, any comments or accounts of action taken (see Table 5.1).

These and other questions are used to formulate the student evaluation placement questionnaire. This should be viewed as a positive quality assurance process but sometimes some students' destructive comments cause staff to feel angry and question why they should make such an effort when students don't appreciate what mentorship entails from the mentor's perspective. Pearce (2007) offers a useful 'ten steps to staff motivation' and

TABLE 5.1   *RCN factors for students to consider whilst on placement*

- You were encouraged by the mentor and the team to evaluate the learning experience both formally or informally.
- You completed the documentation.
- You felt adequately prepared for the practice experience by the HEI.
- The time allocated for the placement was satisfactory to achieve the required competencies and learning outcomes for your stage in the programme.
- The mentor system provided effective support to meet your learning needs.
- The mentor was approachable and enthusiastic about their role within the practice setting.
- You knew how to change mentors if the relationship was not working.
- The placement experience offered you a quality learning experience where safe and effective care was evident.
- This was a satisfactory learning experience.
- There was an opportunity to reflect on this practice placement and the learning experiences within the classroom.
- You were able to meet with your personal tutor to discuss this practice placement.

sometimes it may be necessary for mentors to defuse the anger that they may feel following receiving negative student evaluation comments and counteract those with the positive, rewarding and constructive feedback from others. The motivation that is needed to undertake effective mentorship is identified, valued and respected by the majority of healthcare students and this is the positive stance that should dominate the mentor's commitment to their role and to ensuring that the quality of their practice placement is maintained.

Discuss the quality of the learning environment

There are a number of approaches to gaining information regarding the effectiveness of the learning environment that involve patients, clients, service users, healthcare students as well as those who manage the practice placement. Evaluations are therefore obtained from more than just healthcare students. Mentors have to be aware of the mechanisms for receiving feedback from those patients who receive healthcare or their families, friends and carers. There are a number of supportive mechanisms that monitor the patient healthcare experience and to whom they can provide feedback. A Patient Advisory and Liaison Service is available so that the patient's evaluation of their care can be discussed with someone who is objective.

If patients don't want to directly speak to someone if they have a complaint or wish to offer positive, complimentary comments about their healthcare journey, and those professionals that have contributed at the different stages, they may want to complete a 'patient's opinions count' form that will be sent to the Chief Executive. If the patient has enclosed their name and address, they will receive a direct response that their complaint is being investigated. However, if there is no name but the ward and hospital stated, the complaint will be sent directly to the Directorate Manager to investigate.

Mentors therefore receive evaluation feedback comments about the quality of their learning environment from those who are directly receiving the healthcare services and also from students who are contributing to the delivery of that care, under their guidance. Patients comment not only on the quality of their care but also on the effectiveness of the healthcare professionals' communication and interpersonal skills. As patients need educating about their condition, their altered pathophysiology and why they are experiencing the symptoms that they are, as well as rehabilitation, then a number of strategies should be employed to ensure that transference of knowledge. Patients and relatives reflect on the effectiveness or lack of information within healthcare settings. Although practice placements provide information resources – posters, leaflets, booklets, etc., some areas are more effective than others. Students will be involved in this delivery of health promotion to patients and they gain an insight of patient's expectations and subsequent misconceptions. Evaluation can therefore be viewed as an integral role of being a registered practitioner as well as being a mentor, and is pertinent to all nurses, midwives and allied professions.

The Health Professions Council in their 'Standards of proficiency' clearly identifies the importance of critical evaluation of the impact of, or response to, the registrant's actions.

2c.1: Registrants must be able to monitor and review the ongoing effectiveness of planned activity and modify it accordingly:

- be able to gather information, including qualitative and quantitative data, that helps to evaluate the responses of patients, clients and users to their care;
- be able to evaluate management plans against treatment milestones using recognized health outcome measures and revise the plans as necessary in conjunction with the patient, client or user;
- recognize the need to monitor and evaluate the quality of practice and the value of contributing to the generation of data for quality assurance and improvement programmes;
- be able to make reasoned decisions to initiate, continue, modify or cease treatment or the use of techniques or procedures, and record the decisions and reasoning appropriately (HPC, 2007c; 2007f).

As well as these generic statements, there are some specific requirements according to the individual profession:

- understand that outcomes may not always conform to expectations but may still meet the needs of patients, clients or users (HPC, 2004);
- be able to work in appropriate partnership with the service user in order to evaluate the effectiveness of occupational therapy intervention (HPC, 2007d);
- be able to evaluate treatment plans to ensure that they meet the physiotherapy needs of service users, informed by changes in circumstances and health status (HPC, 2007e).

There is a close proximity of generic variables that can be applied to all healthcare professionals. The success of the interprofessional team work will ensure that patients and their families, friends or carers receive the most effective holistic care that corresponds to their healthcare requirements. The quality of the learning environment may be related to the 'vision' that the professionals have for their specific practice placement.

This is undoubtedly problematic when bombarded by evaluations from healthcare students about the placement and the 'patient's opinions count'. Clark (2008) highlights how this may be a challenge for managers in executing their leadership skills. 'The process of identifying and developing a vision can be demanding because it requires new possibilities to be identified. Individuals who embark on this process are challenging themselves and others to make these possibilities a reality', states Clark (ibid.: 34). In order to respond to the evaluations and develop a vision for future developments of the practice placements, staff are also involved in and have to respond to the process of educational audits.

Educational audits

Mentors may be involved in the audit process from different dimensions. Their contributions are valued as they complete, or assist in the completion of, the audit documentation. They may actually be more involved during the educational audit practice placement visit, talking to the auditors, showing them around the placement or by facilitating the process. All the practice environments that healthcare students are allocated to must have undergone an educational audit in order for that area to be deemed a suitable placement.

According to Marquis and Huston (2006), an audit can be viewed as a systematic and official examination of an environment, hence the practice placement. The process provides feedback to the manager, placement staff and higher education institutions that the set criteria stated in the educational audit document are being adhered to. Marquis and Huston identify three main stages:

1   The criterion or standard is determined.
2   Information is collected to determine if the standard has been met.
3   Educational or corrective action is taken if the criterion has not been met.

The following are the various stages of the educational audit process:

- Establish control criteria – the required standards.
- Identify the information relevant to the criteria – include in audit document.
- Determine ways to collect the information.
- Collect and analyse the information.
- Compare collected information with the established criteria.
- Make a judgement about quality.
- Provide information and, if necessary, take corrective action regarding findings to appropriate sources.
- Re-evaluation (Marquis and Huston, 2006).

Although the process may vary according to individual higher education institutes, the overall audit process could follow a logical sequence. The importance of this awareness is that mentors appreciate the process and how they can contribute accordingly to maintaining an effective learning environment. This awareness may form part of discussions within the Mentor Preparation Courses so that all staff can value how they could make an input.

Educational audit tool – an example

The tool could be designed to provide the criteria for placement staff to answer a series of questions based on the following areas:

* Practice Placement Details – name, address, contact person, the number of students and their grades that the placement is suitable for.
* Reason for the audit must be stated: new placement, annual monitoring, interim review, etc.
* Staff profile: name, job title, hours worked, Nursing/Midwifery/Professional Qualifications.
* An overall descriptive summary of the practice placement.

The audit tool could be designed to focus on a number of specific areas and questions in order to provide the feedback required. For example:

* *Placement safety*: How effectively does the practice placement provide a safe environment for healthcare students?
* *Educational provision*: Are there any appropriate learning opportunities for students in the practice placement?
* *Student support*: Is there evidence of appropriate support for students in the practice placement?
* *Mentorship*: Do students have an appropriately qualified named mentor to provide professional support?
* *Nursing care*: Is the care provided in the practice placement client centred and reflects the rights of clients?

Throughout the audit tool the content relates to outcome audit (end result of care), process audit (process of care) and structure audit (relationship between quality care and appropriate structure) as described by Marquis and Huston (2006). The content clearly relates to a number of mentorship issues, it could provide a culture for self-assessment and encouraging personal reflection on the five identified questions, and an overall evaluation of the effectiveness of the practice placement in the facilitation of student learning.

Educational audit procedure – an example

The mechanism for undertaking any audit procedure is established according to local education and nursing needs. Whatever process is adopted, evaluative feedback needs to be obtained and returned to a centralized area so that the resultant data can be examined, explored and discussed. The following is an example of one method to consider what may be very different from that associated with your local higher educational institute, so you will need to identify how your audit procedure works.

1   Return of completed self-assessment audit document: In order for an educational audit to be undertaken the document is sent to the identified Named Contact Person so that they can complete the questions associated with the five standards; the mentor can offer support if they feel they can. If they have any concerns or wish clarification of any questions, they can contact their educational link for guidance and support. Sometimes the audit document may be completed and returned by an electronic process. Whichever process, the completed document is returned to the higher education institute in preparation to give to the two auditors, who may be a lecturer and a non-related placement staff member. The lecturer tends to take the lead and arranges a mutually agreed date and time for all concerned.

2   Preparation for the audit visit:

   (a)   The two auditors need to check that the documentation is complete and if the required information has been given.
   (b)   If there is any information missing, this can be obtained on the day of visit, otherwise the details need to be checked and areas of concerns identified.
   (c)   It may be appropriate to read the last audit report in case there were any areas identified that needed amending; the changes need to be discussed during the visit.
   (d)   The rationale for the audit visit must be viewed as a positive evaluation strategy that will help to enhance the partnership between the practice placement and the higher education institute.

3   Undertaking an audit visit:

   (a)   This should be viewed as a positive opportunity for the placement staff to express any concerns that may involve any students, their training or assessment strategies to ensure their knowledge is updated.
   (b)   The auditors can have a look around the placement, discuss any issues that arise and offer support or guidance if required.
   (c)   The completed audit document can be discussed, any aspects examined and areas further explored if necessary.
   (d)   The auditors can examine each of the audit questions and discuss any aspects that were documented as a concern on a previous visit.

(e) The intention is to review the role of the mentorship team and discuss areas of support that are available.

(f) If possible the auditors could talk to any students to ensure that they are satisfied with the practice placement.

(g) An initial written feedback report could be given to the staff and any areas that are a concern have to be addressed in an action plan stating the date by which these have to be achieved.

4 Following the audit visit:

(a) The audit report will be finalized, sent to the appropriate audit lead or the placement manager.

(b) If there are any serious issues related to unsafe practice, the auditors have to recommend that any students should be removed and relocated elsewhere.

(c) The practice placement will be taken 'off line' as a recognized suitable environment until the area of concern has been resolved and a follow-up audit is undertaken.

Therefore, mentors do need to understand the importance of the two-year cycle of audits. Year one is the formal audit visit, year two the placement staff undertake their own audit completing the documentation appropriately. This will then be sent to the audit team to be ratified unless there are any identified areas of concern. If these are identified, another formal visit will be arranged otherwise this will complete the two-year cycle. Mentors do play a vital role throughout the process and contribute effectively in order to ensure that this evaluation of practice placement learning and learning opportunities enhances their particular educational profile.

Now complete Mentor Activity 5.3 in order to update your own awareness and to clarify how your practice placement has responded to their last audit visit.

MENTOR ACTIVITY 5.3

Examine your practice placement's last educational audit, familiarize yourself with the content of the audit tool and the final auditors' report.

Within domain four, the NMC (2008a) advocates the importance of mentors appreciating and contributing to the process of evaluation. This is also emphasized by the Health Professions Council (see Table 5.2).

TABLE 5.2   *HPC recommendations for audit*

Section 2c.2 be able to audit, reflect on and review practice

- understand the principles of quality control and quality assurance
- be aware of the role of audit and review in quality management, including quality control, quality assurance and the use of appropriate outcome measures
- be able to maintain an effective audit trail and work towards continual improvement
- participate in quality assurance programmes, where appropriate
- understand the value of reflection on practice and the need to record the outcome of such reflection
- recognize the value of case conferences and other methods of review (HPC, 2004; 2007e; 2007f).

Despite the generic recommendations there are some specific ones such as:

- be able to evaluate nutritional and dietetic information critically, and to engage in the process of reflection in order to inform dietetic practice
- be able to adapt dietetic practice as a result of unexpected outcomes or further information gained during the dietetic intervention (HPC, 2007c)
- be able to recognize the potential of occupational therapy in new and emerging areas of practice (HPC, 2007d)

The importance of undertaking educational audits is therefore pertinent to all healthcare professionals in an attempt to review the effectiveness of the practice placement for facilitating learning for students. There are a number of ways that evaluative feedback is obtained and used as evidence in the establishment of an effective quality assurance process.

Implementing appropriate changes

The significance of undertaking an evaluation is to identify any areas of weaknesses and the need to implement change to improve the learning environment for mentors and healthcare students. There are a number of specific support mechanisms implemented in various universities: these are two examples:

- Practice Learning Teams or equivalent
- Learning Community Education Adviser/Mentor Support Practitioner.

Practice Learning Teams – Teams of Practice and Academic Staff

Practice Learning Teams (PLT) or equivalent were introduced as the result of an investigation into the role of the Link Teacher within placements as it was apparent that this varied according to specific teachers, the time they spent in the practice environment and the role they executed whilst in that role. The feedback from practitioners, teachers and students identified that there were areas of concern and inequality so it was decided to introduce the Practice Learning Team as a possible replacement. Although this or its equivalent named is pertinent to some practice placements, you may have a similar process but, irrespective of its title, the support that is or could be offered needs to be acknowledged and valued. Consider the following and contrast with your practice placement educational support.

The aims of the Practice Learning Team are to do the following:

- Develop effective partnerships between the School of Nursing and the practice areas.
- Reflect a valuing and development of practice-based learning, which is an essential component of the students' learning experience.
- Support practice staff as they facilitate students' learning and achievement of their learning outcomes and competencies through effective assessment processes.

There are a number of PLTs that correspond to the range of specialist areas of nursing and midwifery, comprise both academic representatives as well as from placement and meet on a regular basis. The importance of these meetings are that they provide an appropriate forum to discuss both academic and practice placements changes, student behaviour and the way forward. All student evaluation of placement summaries are presented to the PLT representative so that they can distribute them to their own staff; any areas of concern can then be discussed within the group if appropriate. These teams are viewed as a supportive partnership that offers help to support mentors and other practice placement staff to ensure that the mentorship process is as effective as it can possibly be. The underpinning philosophy behind such teams is to ensure that a more effective working relationship between practice placement staff and educational staff is established, each valuing each other's role and thereby attempting to reduce the alleged and much debated theory–practice gap.

Learning Community Advisers/The Mentor Support Practitioner/ The Practice Support Teacher

Elcock and Sookhoo (2007) stated that there have been a number of concerns expressed regarding the quality of mentorship in supporting pre-registration nursing students in their practice placements. Subsequently, they identify specific areas of concern that have been researched including:

- conflicting demands on mentors between supporting students and caring for patients;
- ineffective preparation for the role of being a mentor;
- lack of understanding of the student's role in practice;
- lack of understanding of the student's training programme.

These are a few examples of the many variables that have been explored and subsequently identified that although mentors do undertake their role as best they can, perhaps a little more support would enhance their effectiveness. Elcock and Sookhoo emphasize the importance of some of these concerns with particular reference to the expectation that students on registration will be fit for practice at the point of registration (Moore, 2005). Therefore, a number of new posts have been introduced: Practice Education Facilitators, Practice Educators, Clinical Placement Facilitators (Jowett and McMullan, 2007), Mentor Support Practitioner, Practice Support Teacher – these are all supportive roles whose remit is to support the mentor and are ultimately linked to the evaluation of the effectiveness of the Making a Difference curriculum (DH, 1999). Irrespective of the specific title, where the role has been introduced, the support offered to the mentors is invaluable.

The Mentor Support Practitioner (MSP) and Practice Support Teacher are examples of these new roles. The MSP is still linked to practice as well as working on a part-time basis within the School of Nursing and whose roles and responsibilities include:

- contributing to the preparation of new mentors;
- introducing the most recent NMC mentorship guidelines;
- helping to support mentors in the practice setting, offering support and guidance as required;
- delivering mentor updates (NMC, 2008a) to groups and on a face-to-face basis;
- offering advice and guidance to students regarding their mentorship experiences.

Although the role of the MSP is continually evolving, there is nevertheless an acknowledgement that mentors do need to be supported as much as they feel is required. The MSP is in the unique and valued position of being able to closely link practice and education. Mentors may have the advantage of working with someone in one of these new roles, how these will change in the future will need to be monitored.

As a result of evaluations, students' feedback is acknowledged and any areas of concern are discussed with mentors, members of the Practice Learning Team or the Mentor Support Practitioner as a contemporary approach to ensuring the practice provides appropriate learning opportunities for all the healthcare students undertaking a placement experience.

The NMC (2008e) *Prep Handbook* offers a series of interesting case studies and scenarios for you to reflect on.

Frequently asked questions

Mentors

Q. What is the point of students completing a placement evaluation when all they ever do is criticize and say hurtful things about the staff? Don't students realize we came into nursing to 'nurse', mentorship is something extra that we are involved in, in order to ensure that our practice area is recognized for the potential that it does have to offer?

A. All students' evaluation of placements should be viewed in an objective manner and mentors must try to ascertain the meaning of the actual or inferred comments. Evaluation is an important aspect of quality assurance but it is also acknowledged that unjustifiable negative comments must be viewed with caution.

Q. The practice placement self-audit document was completed by our manager and only a select few staff members were involved. I thought that mentors had a more valued contribution to the completion of the practice placement audit?

A. The completion of the self-audit document is undertaken by placement staff before an academic audit visit. The document is a summary that reflects what your placement has to offer including the ratio of mentors to students, the training and recent updates undertaken by the identified mentors. In some practice placements staff do make a more involved contribution than in other areas but this decision is up to the overall manager to orchestrate.

Students

Q. What is the point of completing a student evaluation of placement if the problems I had, other students state they have experienced the same? Why do some mentors continue to mentor even though they have a very poor, negative and anti-student reputation?

A. There are a number of reasons why health professionals undertake the mentorship training and subsequent role. These can be professional and viewed as an integral requirement for the job that they undertake. Their professional accountability is dependent on their commitment to mentorship. They are now working towards completing their triennial review requirements whereby they have to mentor at least two in a three-year period (NMC, 2008a). On a personal level they may see this as an attempt to feel that they are a contributing team member who is respected, valued and proactive. Unfortunately, there is a dichotomy between the mentor's perception and the student, who is the receiver of this mentorship experience.

Q. My colleague and I started the same placement, same time, same week but unfortunately by week two we were both very upset and distressed by the negative approach shown by our mentors. The situation became worse as we were 'told' by the mentors that they were having difficulty finding time to teach us, so they suggested we spent our time in the School library and updated their 'Student Welcoming Pack!' How does that justify our adult branch experience?

A. Unfortunately this situation emphasizes that sometimes mentors do have difficulty balancing all their roles and responsibilities associated with being a leader, manager and teacher. Although there is an irony in what you were asked to do, the situation could have been utilized effectively. However, if students are concerned about what they are asked to do in the practice placement, they must discuss their concerns with the mentor, placement, manager, academic link or personal tutor.

Chapter summary

This chapter has focused on the process of evaluation as a means of gaining feedback from healthcare students regarding their practice placement experience. Having completed this chapter you have learned about:

* the process of evaluation, the types of evaluations that healthcare students have to complete, particularly their evaluation of placement;
* the quality of student's comments is valued as part of the quality assurance mechanism but caution has to be made in order to identify evaluation bias;
* mechanisms for gaining feedback from students regarding the mentorship process, the learning resources, the mentor and the quality of the practice placement;

- the importance of practice placement completing the self-audit document and the importance of an audit visit as a reciprocal support mechanism;
- the importance of evaluative feedback as the process for identifying and developing further aspects of learning in order to enhance the effectiveness of the practice placement.

Further reading

Nursing and Midwifery Council (NMC) (2008e) The Prep Handbook. London: NMC.

This is an updated version of the previous guidelines and includes examples of Prep (CPD) learning based on 17 case studies in five different healthcare specialities including: Acute care, Midwifery, Community care, Education and research, Management and Practising in other areas. The case studies explore a description and the outcome of learning activities, and examine how the learning activity relates to the individual's workplace.

6

What makes an 'effective' placement for healthcare students?

David Kinnell

The Nursing and Midwifery Council (2008a): Eight domains of mentorship
Domain Five: Creating an environment for learning

Aim

Create an environment for learning, where practice is valued and developed, that provides appropriate professional and interprofessional learning opportunities and support for learning to maximize achievement for individuals.

Outcomes

Stage 1: Nurses and Midwives

- Demonstrate a commitment to continuing professional development to enhance own knowledge and proficiency.
- Provide peer support to others to facilitate their learning.

Stage 2: Mentor

- Support students to identify both learning needs and experiences that are appropriate to their level of learning.
- Use a range of learning experiences, involving patients, clients, carers and the professional team, to meet defined learning needs.
- Identify aspects of the learning environment which could be enhanced negotiating with others to make appropriate changes.
- Act as a resource to facilitate personal and professional development of others.

Introduction

The practice placement should provide the ideal environment for mentors to encourage healthcare students to relate theory to practice (Koh, 2002; RCN, 2004; 2007b). Most training programmes start the course with an exploration of significant theory that will enhance the student's understanding and awareness of the healthcare experience that is pertinent to both the profession and the classification of patient that they will be caring for once the introductory period is complete. Students are exposed to an idealistic stance of healthcare whilst in the classroom environment and working in the practice placement allows the opportunity to relate this idealism to reality, irrespective of profession.

It is envisaged that a general approach to exploring the effectiveness of the practice placement will be the main focus of this chapter, so that the content will maintain an interprofessional approach and be relevant to healthcare students: midwives, nurses, as well as other related health professions. However, it would be useful to start with a review of the NMC's (2008a) domain five as a number of factors are pertinent to all healthcare professionals.

What makes an 'effective' learning environment?

The Nursing and Midwifery Council (2004c) requires that pre-registration programmes are appropriately designed to ensure there is an even division in time spent between studying theory and then applying that knowledge into practice. Therefore, the role of the mentor is instrumental in meeting those statutory requirements. Indeed, the Royal College of Nursing (2007b: 1) states: 'As a mentor you have the privilege and responsibility of helping students translate theory into practice and making reality of what is learned in the classroom.' It is a role that is challenging but nevertheless can be extremely rewarding.

The healthcare environment varies from the traditional National Health Service hospital and community settings to those related to the voluntary and independent sector, all contributing experience to the patient, client or service user throughout their healthcare journey. The student will be able to access an insight into both short stay and long stay healthcare experiences and value the importance of interprofessional contributions made by all allied professions. There is no doubt that there is a marked dichotomy between some healthcare students' perception of healthcare and the experience that they are actually exposed to.

Therefore, it would be useful for all mentors to complete Mentor Activity 6.1 before contrasting your views with that of student nurses.

MENTOR ACTIVITY 6.1

Reflect on your own personal and professional experiences whilst answering the following question.

'What makes an effective placement for healthcare students?'
Make some notes before proceeding with this chapter.

This is a thought-provoking mentor activity which will help you to review your own placement area and ascertain the potential and actual opportunities that it may provide for healthcare students. The mentor needs to capitalize on these in order to enhance the learning experience for students and fulfil the requirements within this NMC (2008a) domain.

Reflecting on Mentor Activity 6.1, a number of third-year student nurses (from 2003–2008) as part of a management lesson classroom activity were asked the same question and a summary of their responses is presented in Box 6.1. Although a number of different cohorts were involved, there were a number of similar responses.

Box 6.1   What makes an 'effective' placement for student nurses?

1   The Placement

- A welcoming atmosphere.
- An effective working team.
- To be recognized as someone who wants to learn.
- Placements that are informed and prepared for student's arrival.
- Not being treated as an 'extra pair of hands'.
- Working as part of the multi-disciplinary team.
- Being introduced to patients and other staff members.
- Being given responsibility to develop.

2   Mentorship

- Mentors who know their student's name and not refer to them as 'the student'.
- A mentor who wants to mentor.

(Continued)

(Continued)

- Mentors whose knowledge is up to date.
- An enthusiastic and supportive mentor.
- Mentors who help students complete their placement booklet.
- Regular feedback from mentors on students' progress.
- Mentors who don't keep swapping their shifts without telling their student, when previously arranged to work together.
- Helping students achieve their practice competencies.

3   Availability of resources:

- Availability of learning resources.
- Appropriate teaching sessions.
- Being encouraged to use available resources for personal and professional development without being made to feel 'guilty'.
- The opportunity to visit other clinical areas, and encouraged to do so.

What makes an 'effective' placement for students? The practice placement

It is during this experiential exposure that students develop their perception of the reality of how their chosen health profession contributes to the patients', residents', users' or carers' healthcare experience. It is an anticipated resultant end product of this experience that the effectiveness of communication and interpersonal skills will be challenged. Therefore, the comments highlighted by the third-year student nurses stated in the Mentor Activity 6.1 could also be echoed by other healthcare students as part of the multi-disciplinary team experience. A 'welcoming atmosphere' and an 'effective team' may have different connotations to different students but predominantly the importance of team cohesion and a feeling of belongingness are central to gaining the most from any healthcare placements.

The English National Board for Nursing and Midwifery and the Department of Health (ENB/DH) (2001) explored the significance and variation in practice placements in their document *Placements in Focus*. They provided a useful checklist that placement staff could use in order to audit and evaluate their own contributions and success story. The checklist is divided into four sections, each encouraging a different interlocking variable to be explored, and can be used as guidance to ascertain good practice. The series of questions identifies issues that have to be considered in the planning, provision and evaluation of practice placement experiences, based around the four headings:

1 Providing practice placements
2 Practice learning environment
3 Student support
4 Assessment of practice.

TABLE 6.1   *The practice learning environment*

1	Does the practice area have a stated philosophy of care which is reflected in practice and supports curriculum aims?
2	Does the practice provision reflect respect for the rights of health service users and their carers?
3	Does the provision of care reflect respect for the privacy, dignity and religious and cultural beliefs and practices of patients and clients?
4	Is care provision based on relevant research-based and evidence-based findings where available?
5	Does care provision involve different models of care commensurate with current practice and encompassing local and national initiatives?
6	Are interpersonal and practice skills fostered through a range of teaching/learning methods?
7	Does the practice experience enable students to experience the role of the registered practitioner in a range of contexts?
8	Do all placements have an infrastructure to support continuing professional development opportunities for practitioners?
9	Do students gain experience as part of a multiprofessional team?
10	Do the sequencing and balance between university and practice-based study promote the integration of knowledge, attitudes and skills?
11	Is a learning resource area available in the practice environment?
12	Does student feedback contribute to the ongoing evaluation of the learning environment and the student experience and are all stakeholders aware of the feedback?
	(ENB/DH, 2001)

The ENB/DH (2001) ask 12 questions in their section focused on the practice learning environment (Table 6.1). As a mentor, it would be advantageous for you to answer the following in order to evaluate the effectiveness of your practice setting and identify any areas that possibly need to be further developed. This would be a useful exercise for all mentors to undertake.

There is no doubt that this checklist is a vital starting point for all mentors who wish to reflect and evaluate the effectiveness of their own associated practice placements, in an attempt to gain a conceptualized vision of healthcare students' experiences. In support, Koh (2002) emphasizes that understanding research–based and evidence-based findings should help students understand and appreciate the relevance of theory to practice. However, for some students, their practice placement may be viewed as a complex experience, so support and guidance from mentors are paramount.

Therefore, an 'effective' placement for healthcare students will depend on the perception of their own personal goals and aspirations. Interestingly, it could be argued that the same practice placement can play host to a number of students at varying stages of their training, and hence the acqui-sition of achievements will be determined by individualized expectations. It is the usual procedure to inform the placement, in the agreed time span, of the proposed allocation of students, level of training, and time they will spend in that setting. The students will arrive expecting that these adminis-trative preparations have been executed. So, it is with some empathy, that the placement staff must appreciate the disappointment that students' expe-rience when they are told that their arrival was unexpected. Sometimes this is a difficult situation to comprehend but nevertheless students do report that this misconception heralded their first encounter of the placement team that they were looking forward to becoming a member of.

Once the orientation programme has been implemented, the student should have met their mentor and or associate/co-mentor. They have had the opportunity to discuss their expectations of the placement and also highlighted what competencies, outcomes or proficiencies they need to achieve. So, first impressions seem to indicate that the interpersonal and practice skills will be fostered as part of that placement experience. Unfortunately, student nurses' personal accounts conversely reveal disap-pointments because they were not valued, their learning aspirations were not acknowledged, and proclaimed incidences of being used as an 'extra pair of hands'. In contrast, students do share accounts of being recognized as someone who wants to learn, develop and be incorporated as part of the working team by being introduced to patients and other staff members. These components accentuate variables of a placement that encourages active participation in the learning process.

From a supporting perspective, the RCN (2007b) provides a useful checklist of recommendations that all healthcare mentors could use to analyse the effectiveness of their practice area, irrespective of the type of student being mentored. This reaffirms factors identified by the ENB/DH (2001). The combination of both checklists should help all mentors appraise the effectiveness of their placement and ascertain to what extent it enhances learning.

The RCN (2007b: 10) states that an effective practice placement should promote learning and help students to do the following:

1   Meet the statutory and regulatory requirements and, where applicable, European directives.
2   Achieve the required learning outcomes and competencies according to regulatory body requirements for pre-registration.
3   Work alongside mentors who are appropriately prepared, creating a partnership with them.
4   Identify appropriate learning opportunities to meet their learning needs.
5   Use their time effectively, creating opportunities to enable the application of theory to practice and vice versa.
6   Work within a wide range of rapidly changing health and social services that recognize the continuing nature of care.
7   Demonstrate an appreciation of the multi-professional approach to care.
8   Maintain their supernumerary status.

The importance of exploring these two checklists and examining the student nurses' perspective will allow mentors to examine to what extent their own practice placement meets these guidelines. If there are any areas of weakness or any deficits, hopefully you will consider how to improve those areas discovered. Mentor Activity 6.2 will encourage you to reflect on what your environment has to offer to healthcare students and any potential areas for future development.

MENTOR ACTIVITY 6.2

Examine the RCN (2007b) checklist and examine the effectiveness of your practice placement.

Are there any areas that you think need to be and could be improved?

Whilst in the practice placement, a number of associated underpinning theoretical perspectives can be applied to justify the acquisition of healthcare knowledge. One perspective is that proposed by Bandura (1977) in his 'Social learning theory'. Linking theory to practice, it is anticipated that healthcare students will be encouraged to develop self-empowerment whilst internalizing the knowledge, skills and attitudes pertinent to their health profession.

In order to accentuate this process, students will face the realism encapsulated within the dichotomy whereby practice is not always driven by the most recent evidence or practice-based findings and recommendations. Nevertheless, a proactive practice placement should be a climate in which this apparent disparity can be discussed in order to verify that the apparent knowledge of the staff collectively is updated.

However, read through Case study 6.1 before going on to the next section.

CASE STUDY 6.1

A second-year adult branch student nurse complained to his Personal Tutor about the ward. He stated that his mentor was not supportive and the rest of the staff made him feel that he didn't belong there. This was week three, of a seven-week placement.

Discussing his concerns, it appeared to him that all the nursing staff were at fault. He felt he was not being allowed to develop as the learning opportunities he wanted to access were being restricted to him. He stated that he was mainly involved in the menial tasks that he did when he was in his first year. As a second-year student he wanted to be more involved in wound care, administration of medicines under supervision, and more directly in assessing pre- and post-operative care needs for patients that he was caring for, again under guidance of qualified staff.

Unfortunately, the ward was busy, the staffing level was a problem due to sickness, maternity and annual leave. His main mentor was often in charge of the ward, so he did appreciate she was busy. His associate mentor he had met in week one, and since then, he had been on annual leave. The student had apparently been complaining about his mentor to the other staff. Conversely, he had been complaining to his mentor about the lack of support he had received from the other staff members of the team.

This situation had caused conflict among the staff and what is usually an effective conducive learning environment had been disrupted by this student. The staff felt disappointed that he had 'reported' them to the School of Nursing without clearly discussing his concerns to them.

The ward was well established and had a very positive reputation as a good placement, with various resources and learning opportunities to access. The team of staff are generally very committed to mentorship. At the last audit visit, the findings were positive and the staff were commended on their commitment to creating an environment for learning.

Unfortunately, the experience this student claimed he was going through did raise concerns and highlighted the importance of misconceptions.

How do you think this situation should have been managed and what would you do to ensure that the learning environment was not compromised?

There are a number of ways of dealing with this case study but the most important issue is to remind mentors that all their efforts and contributions to the effectiveness of their placement are valued and appreciated by the majority of healthcare students. Mentors are used to dealing with patient individuality which may be outside the norm at times, and the same consideration may apply to some students. The important consideration for the mentors is that mentorship is a positive two-way professional relationship and although well established, sometimes this may be challenged. However, from all negative experiences there is usually a positive learning end product, so mentors must not take this personally but reflect on the experience and highlight what they have learnt that could be applied in the future.

What makes an 'effective' placement for students?: mentorship

This is important because all qualified staff are in a position to identify, explore and initiate change that could ultimately benefit the delivery of healthcare (Bahn, 2001). However, some staff are content to continue without the pressure of becoming involved in contemporary healthcare debates regarding implementing change based on evidence or research findings. In reality, therefore, students may be exposed to dynamic, proactive and abstract thinking mentors or conversely, one who is more of a traditionalist, concrete-thinker who is content with pre-existing, established healthcare policies and procedures. The student's perception and final evaluation of that allocated practice placement will therefore be influenced by the type of mentorship that they are exposed to.

Bandura (1977) explored this experiential exposure concept and encapsulated the underpinning ideology within his social learning theory. Associated with the well-established psychological concept and learning theory of behaviourism, social learning theory amalgamates understanding of the individual's observable overt behaviour and the way that they think. Therefore, Bandura (1977) proposed the 'cognitive-behavioural' approach which emphasizes the inter-relationship between the way we think (cognitivism) and the behaviour (behaviourism) that is displayed during any social interaction. This effectively relates to the professional relationship between the healthcare student and the patient, client or service user. The effectiveness of this inter-relationship could be attributed to the vicarious learning, the process of learning without realizing that learning is taking place, which is an inherent result in the process of role modelling.

Bandura's (1977) theory highlights the dynamic influence of observing other people's behaviour and adopting now or in the future, aspects of that observed learning. In contemporary healthcare, students are allocated to practice placements in order to observe the behaviour and interactions between them and those that they are delivering aspects of care to. The mentor is therefore a significant linchpin in helping students to learn acceptable healthcare behaviour that they can further develop. However, although the principle of role modelling is to expose the student to observing professionals, experience in the practice placement can be attributed not only acquiring clinical skills but also to gaining an awareness of professional attitudes and effective interactions between patients and members of the multi-disciplinary team. Unfortunately, this may have a negative end result.

It is hoped that the influence of social learning, role modelling and experiential learning will be positive, contrived and advantageous to the development of the learner. However, there is no scope for complacency as some reflective accounts from students do differentiate between an effective proactive placement and one in which their reflective memories are predominantly negative. Bahn (2001) emphasizes that students not only want to 'fit in' as part of the placement team, they have to identify the ideal role model, the professional that would like to emulate in their future careers. Students hopefully develop their knowledge, skills and attitudes throughout their training journey as they aspire to internalize the components that combine to produce the ideal healthcare professional. Therefore, it could be argued that a combination of an effective learning environment, a proactive mentor who is acknowledged as an ideal role model and a motivated student, should be the prerequisites to guaranteeing an effective training journey for healthcare students.

Furthermore, Bandura (1986) asserts that role modelling is an effective vehicle that allows the mentor the opportunity to transfer cognitive intrapersonal functions of values, beliefs, attitudes and aspirations. However, he emphasizes that simple 'imitation' will not be productive to encourage student learning – the process is more complex. Healthcare experience from the student's perspective is an attempt to relate theory to care delivery whilst working in a practice placement. Role modelling is a more intricate process that incorporates the four dimensions (see Box 6.2) of attentional processes, retention processes, motor reproduction processes and motivational processes (Bahn, 2001; Donaldson and Carter, 2005; Quinn and Hughes, 2007).

Box 6.2   The four-dimensional model of role modelling

Attentional Processes + Retention Processes + Motor Preproduction Processes + Motivation = Role Modelling

Attentional processes associated with role modelling

Bandura (1986) differentiates between the characteristics of the role model and those of the observer – mentor and student. The feedback from the mentor, positive and negative, verbal and non-verbal will have a resultant impact on the student. The process of learning is not merely enhanced by exposure to the subject focus but requires some response as part of a feedback mechanism. Positive reinforcement for desired behaviour demonstrated by the mentor will ensure that the associated modelled healthcare behaviour will be acknowledged by the student. However, the effectiveness will depend on the psychological functional processes of that student including their ability to process learned information, their perceptual abilities and previous experiences within the learning process.

Mentors identify the different capabilities of students to learn and develop their knowledge, skills and professional attitudes as dependent on the individual's interest, willingness to learn and appreciation of the experience observed as part of the patient's healthcare journey. However, some aspects of care delivery, healthcare procedures, and promoting self-care managements for some patients may need to be observed on more than one occasion, in order for the student to fully internalize, retain and be able to reproduce the behaviour demonstrated. This forms a valued foundation within the mentor and student professional relationship.

Retention processes associated with role modelling

For students, the process of retention of knowledge is paramount in order for them to be able to demonstrate transferable skills from one healthcare setting to another. For example, from a hospital setting to a community-based placement visiting individuals in their own homes, or in a nursing home/care centre. Bahn (2001) clearly emphasizes the importance of being able to relate conceptual ideological discussions into the reality of care delivery and management. Practical procedures are demonstrated and practised in higher educational institutes, in classroom settings or clinical skills laboratories before the student actually applies that procedure to a recipient of healthcare services. Hence, this offers a rationale for the use of OSCEs (Objective Structured/Simulation Clinical Examinations) (NMC, 2008a) as a means of exposing students to potential healthcare situations before they actually arrive at the practice placement or to reflect on the knowledge, skills and attitudes developed whilst they were in the healthcare environment.

Bandura (1977) suggests that students consider the process of coding as a mechanism in assisting their process of retention, a suggestion that may be useful for mentors too. A number of effective strategies are used including acronyms, a word made from a series of initial letters or parts of words. A familiar acronym when reviewing the effectiveness of the communication process for all healthcare students is SOLER (Egan, 2007). This represents:

S–sit squarely whilst talking to the patient, client or service user;

O–open posture should be adopted, being careful with the non-verbal message being relayed;

L–leaning slightly forward to convey interest without invading the other person's body space;

E–eye contact should be maintained;

R–relaxed, indicating that you are interested in what the other person is saying.

These types of acronyms can be useful in assisting learning whilst in the practice placement and can be further developed according to the feedback they receive from their mentor (Donaldson and Carter, 2005).

Gross (2005) explores the fundamental process of learning and memory, emphasizing that this function is a series of three stages (Box 6.3). This theory has implications for understanding the student's learning process in the practice placement and is useful for mentors to reflect on their own learning process.

Box 6.3   The process of memory

- Encoding
- Storage
- Retrieval

Memory Stage One – encoding
This relates to the processes that occur during the presentation of learning material. Whilst in the practice placement healthcare students encounter a myriad of information about patients, their condition, investigations, treatments, management and rehabilitation. The mentor's role is to present the information so that the student can understand the underpinning theoretical perspectives and relate them to the individual patient, client, or service user receiving healthcare.

In order that a practice placement can be recognized by students as an area that is an effective learning environment, dynamic, research- and evidence-based, a number of resources and teaching sessions have to be established and delivered that will help the student to learn from that educational discourse. The effectiveness of encoding is determined on how the medical jargon is presented to the student, ensuring that it is not difficult to comprehend for junior students, but stimulating enough for more senior ones. The mentor will explain the aspects of the patient's journey and the interrelatedness of the interprofessional team of allied health professionals at an educational level that will assist the student to internalize the information.

Memory Stage Two – storage
This is the result of encoding the presented information in a manner that results in positive learning. The student will store the information until such time as it can be applied to practice whilst the role of the mentor is to assist with this process. In order to maintain that data, the student will need to re-visit what has been encoded and maintain its currency. This can be achieved by:

- question and answer sessions with the mentor and other placement staff;
- reflective discussions based on actual or potential healthcare scenarios;
- reflective writing to summarize application of theory to practice;
- simulation exercises to enact potential healthcare emergencies, for example,
- using manikins to represent a patient suffering a cardiac arrest.

These sources of evidence, relating theory to practice, will enable the student to ascertain the effectiveness of their learning and identify with their mentor areas of uncertainty that need further development.

Memory Stage Three – retrieval
This is the process of recovering stored information from the memory system. The effectiveness of the encoding and storage will be evident when the healthcare student starts applying their understanding to the actual delivery of healthcare, undertaking procedures according to those previously demonstrated and being able to discuss the relevant research or evidence pertinent to that practiced with their mentor. The positive reputation of the practice placement can be attributed to the effectiveness, motivation and encouragement given to healthcare students by that established placement team and particularly their valued mentor. The student must discuss their learning needs with their mentor, who, in response, will encourage

that positive response. The mentor therefore makes a valuable and effective contribution to the student's ability to remember and apply theory to practice whilst delivering healthcare.

Retrieval is also related to the ability of the student to associate the information delivered, explored and discussed in the classroom setting to the reality of actual patient presentational features within the healthcare setting. It is anticipated that as the student continues throughout their training journey, the experience gained will be collected into a repertoire of useful theory and practice that they can use as a baseline for further development once gaining their registration. Therefore, mentors have a role in helping students with their development throughout their training that will enhance the knowledge, skills and attitudes in readiness for the continuity of lifelong learning. Hence, Bandura's Social Learning component of retention is of significant importance to all mentors who reflect on the effectiveness of their own learning environments.

Motor reproduction processes associated with role modelling

Throughout a healthcare student's training journey they may be assessed on a number of occasions to ensure that they can reproduce what they have been taught and demonstrated. Quinn and Hughes (2007: 99) state: 'The learner must be capable of actually carrying out the observed behaviour and of evaluating it in terms of accuracy.' Use of the OSCEs is only one assessment strategy that attempts to use simulation in order to assess whether practical skills have been learnt and can be demonstrated when required whilst caring for patients.

Both Bahn (2001) and Donaldson and Carter (2005) emphasize that it may not be until the healthcare student has qualified, that they truly reproduce the practical skills that they have acquired. However, there does appear to be some inconsistencies between which skills mentors demonstrate, and the ones that they will allow the student to carry out. There seems to be a lack of trust on the part of some mentors, often justifiable, which is evident in the restrictive delivery of healthcare they allow students to master. This can certainly be related to student nurses who return from their first placements with descriptions of the wide range of nursing interventions that their mentor demonstrated and allowed them to practise under supervision. Conversely, some student's reflective accounts are not as vigorous with enthusiasm and positive feedback, leading to feelings of envy from their colleagues. The role of the mentor is to maintain their accountability and follow the guidelines within the Code (NMC, 2008b; van der Gaag, 2008). This will subsequently have an impact on the final component within Bandura's (1977) social learning theory.

Motivation associated with role modelling

During discussions of mentorship, mentors attending their yearly mentor update often comment that they are surprised by the extent of motivation in some students and, conversely, the apparent lack of it in others. There are a number of potential reasons for this apparent disparity in student behaviour. Unfortunately, working in a practice placement may not actually meet the idealistic expectations that students have created in their hypothetical vision of what healthcare practice actually entails. It is disappointing when mentors report negative feedback regarding a student's apparent lack of interest and motivation, particularly when it is their first practice placement. The underlying causative factor for this apparent lack of motivation is the dichotomy between idealism and reality.

Regarding Bandura's (1977) social learning theory, there is also a potential problem when the student's perception of their mentor as a role model is associated with negative connotations. The student may feel that their mentor does not display the professionalism that they anticipated. There is no doubt that some mentors do not 'want' to be a mentor but they are forced into the role in order to advance their own professional development. In some practice placements, there are no negotiations between the student and mentor, they are often paired, as soon as the student commences their placement (Andrews and Chilton, 2000). However, most mentors enjoy their role and the positive contribution to mentorship and find working with students enlightening. However, if there are concerns with students working with their mentor particularly because of time constraints, then this emphasizes the importance of initiating support from an associate or co-mentor.

According to Bahn (2001), there are three elements that encourage a student to perform effectively in practice: external incentives, vicarious reinforcement and self-reflection:

- *External*: External incentives include rewards when the student demonstrates overt or observable behaviour that is an appropriate expectation of the mentor and other members of the placement team. From the student's perspective, because the mentor signs their documentation to verify their achievements (competencies, outcomes or proficiencies), this is in itself the desired reward that the student is aiming to achieve. However, this is not always the situation and for whatever reasons, some students do seem to adopt a negative approach which influences the ineffectiveness of the mentorship. If the student is not interested, the mentor may ask themselves why should they be bothered.
- *Vicarious reinforcements*: According to Bandura (1977), this is the end product of observing others' achievements, both successes and failures. Students complain that no matter what effort they make, they seem to feel that they were not welcome in the practice placement and even worse, the staff didn't want them to be there. Some students claim that they are made to feel more of a hindrance and they 'only

got in the way'. This is often as a result of misconception, a blasé statement that could have been ambiguous. However, when patients, residents or service users make complimentary comments about the student to their mentor, the assumption is that the student must be making an impression and are becoming a valued member of that team. This positive feedback assists the mentor with their assessment of the student's suitability for healthcare.

- *Self-reflection*: Alternatively, students are encouraged to engage in self-reflection as part of their own self-awareness and in order to recognize their own achievements, both in theory and practice. Individual students have their own aspirations and idealistic stance on what they want to achieve whilst working in the practice placement.

    It is interesting to listen to students reflecting on their own individual achievements and those of their colleagues. This often leads to a positive self-evaluation as a reward for the interest and motivation that they displayed whilst in the healthcare setting and the effectiveness of working with a supportive mentor. Unfortunately, this could lead to other students feeling a sense of envy or a reaffirmation of their own negative views compared to their colleagues.

Donaldson and Carter (2005) emphasize that there is a predominant need to have an effective role model in order to reinforce good practice. Some students try to show empathy with the practice placement staff when there is a shortage of mentors or qualified staff due to holidays, sickness, or study leave. Bandura (1986) clearly advocates the importance of an effective role model and the quality of exposure of the student to healthcare experiences, care delivery and management.

What makes an 'effective' placement for students?: Availability of resources

Different healthcare settings are responsible for ensuring their reputation for the effectiveness and dynamic approach that they have towards ensuring that student's learning is enhanced by available resources. Students are encouraged to adopt a student-centred approach and therefore, they are responsible for utilizing the resources available. However, in reality, there is a definite demarcation between a placement that has developed and sustained available resources for students to access and those that do not always see this as a priority because of time constraints, lack of staff motivation, financial implications, and general malaise caused by working conditions where there is staff shortages caused by sickness, holidays, maternity leave, study leave, etc.

When students were able to access resources, sometimes they were made to feel uncomfortable or even guilty for using the practice placement time so effectively from their perspective, but this was not perceived by healthcare professionals in the same way. There are a range of resources that can be collected, amalgamated and developed that could be used by all healthcare staff, not just students. The main problem for some areas is the lack of an identified office, resource or study room which could be used in order to increase the effectiveness of using the resources.

Where this is available, students find the facility worthwhile, positive and reassuring, whilst others don't actually use or appreciate the time and effort that staff have dedicated in establishing this resource area. In some placements, with limited room facilities, there is a dedicated trolley or cupboard for storing some of the resources that can then be taken into the day room or any other appropriate area. The range of resources is not restrictive, it has to be relevant to the speciality of healthcare (Table 6.2).

Also, it is important to arrange and establish: planned programmes on insight visits. Spending time as deemed necessary with nurses, midwives, or

TABLE 6.2   *Range of educational resources*

- *Activity sheets* completed and used by students as evidence of their achievements and development of their practice-based learning

- *Anatomical models* used by the various health professions

- *Books* general: anatomy/physiology; specific: related healthcare according to profession; relevant to level of student: Diploma, Degree, Masters Degree

- *Case studies* to read/include activities to complete

- *Computer programs* (Computer Assisted Learning Programmes)

- *CD-Rom/Internet access*

- *Electronic learning exercises/programmes*

- *Health education information* booklets, leaflets, pamphlets, posters examining and presenting a variety of health promotion activities or information booklets given to patients can also be informative. Also, guidance to electronic health information (NHS Choices, 2008)

- *Journals and magazines* general and specific to individual health profession

- *Medical equipment* access to medical equipment, machinery, etc. to practise with and develop practical skills

- *Prepared PowerPoint presentations* specific focus for health professionals

- *Resource folders/files* general and specific to profession according to identified topics, general principles of healthcare, articles of interest

- *Scenarios* actual or potential healthcare situations for the students to discuss, make notes, and feed back

- *Study days (full or half-day)* Some of these award a Certificate of Attendance

- *Training programme* specific to individual health profession

- *Videos/DVDs* examining and presenting a range of health-related topics

- *Workbooks or worksheets* focus on general or specific topics

- *X-rays* sample radiographs can be useful in order to assist explanation of a patient's condition, and their subsequent deterioration or improvement

members of the allied health professions in order to gain an interprofessional understanding of each other's contribution to the patient's healthcare journey.

The Health Professions Council (2008) states that all health professions must protect the health and well-being of people who use or need their related services. The following is a checklist that is used as basic guidance for a number of health professions including dietitians, occupational therapists, operating department practitioners, physiotherapists, and speech and language therapists, but the data could also be interrelated with nursing and midwifery. As from 1st July 2008, their previous 16 standards of conduct, performance and ethics have been condensed into 14 in order to set out the aims more clearly or to correct any mistakes. The standards are, 'both fit for purpose and reflect both professional and public expectations of the behaviour of registrants' (HPC, 2008). The following are the revised standards:

1   You must act in the best interest of service users.
2   You must respect the confidentiality of service users.
3   You must keep high standards of personal conduct.
4   You must provide (to us and any other relevant regulators) any important information about your conduct and competence.
5   You must keep your professional knowledge and skills up to date.
6   You must act within the limits of your knowledge, skills and experience and, if necessary, refer the matter to another practitioner.
7   You must communicate properly and effectively with service users and other practitioners.
8   You must effectively supervise tasks that you have asked other people to carry out.
9   You must get informed consent to give treatment (except in an emergency).
10 You must keep accurate records.
11 You must deal fairly and safely with the risks of infection.
12 You must limit your work or stop practising if your performance or judgement is affected by your health.
13 You must behave with honesty and integrity and make sure that your behaviour does not damage the public's confidence in you or your profession.
14 You must make sure that any advertising you do is accurate. (HPC, 2008)

There is therefore, a close similarity between the Health Professions Council's checklist (2007b; 2008) and the recommendations advocated by the Nursing and Midwifery Council (2008a). In *The Code: Standards of Conduct, Performance and Ethics for Nurses and Midwives*, the NMC (2008b) highlights four main categories in which a number of subsections are identified:

*   Make the care of people your first concern, treating them as individuals and respecting their dignity.
*   Work with others to protect and promote the health and well-being of those in your care, their families and carers, and the wider community.
*   Provide a high standard of practice and care at all times.
*   Be open and honest, act with integrity and uphold the reputation of your profession.

Although both these Standards of conduct, performance and ethics will have an impact on both mentors and their healthcare students, they will ultimately influence the effectiveness of the practice placement. The Health Professions Council (2007c–f) currently regulates thirteen health professions, in each of their standards there is a generic structure that is pertinent to all health professionals (see Box 6.4).

Box 6.4   The HPC (2007) overall structure

- 1a: Professional autonomy and accountability
- 1b: Professional relationships
- 2a: Identification and assessment of health and social care needs
- 2b: Formulations and delivery of plans and strategies for meeting health and social care needs
- 2c: Critical evaluation of the impact of, or response to, the registrant's actions
- 3: Knowledge, understanding and skills

Section 3 is subdivided into three and section 3a.3 relates to the need to establish and maintain a safe practice environment. A number of recommendations are pertinent for all mentors, nursing, midwifery and allied health professions as they have a generic basis.

The standard of proficiency states that the health professional needs to do the following:

- Be aware of applicable health and safety legislation, and any relevant safety policies and procedures in force at the workplace, such as incident reporting, and be able to act in accordance with these.
- Be able to work safely, including being able to select appropriate hazard control and risk management, reduction or elimination techniques in a safe manner in accordance with health and safety legislation.
- Be able to select appropriate personal protective equipment and use it correctly.
- Be able to establish safe environments for practice, which minimize risks to service users, those treating them, and others, including the use of hazard control and particularly infection control.

There are a number of specific aspects related to individual health professions:

- Be able to advise on safe procedures for food preparation – dietitians (HPC, 2007c).
- Know and be able to apply appropriate moving and handling techniques – occupational therapists (HPC, 2007d); physiotherapists (HPC, 2007e).
- Understand the nature and purpose of sterile fields, and the practitioner's individual role and responsibility for maintaining them.
- Understand and be able to apply appropriate moving and handling techniques – operating department practitioners (HPC, 2004).

Throughout the practice placements students will be supported by their mentor and be given the opportunity to discuss their progress and how they feel about the experience gained in order to avoid some of the questions identified in the previous section. The mentor will have given the student feedback at an initial, intermediate and as part of the final interview. This will allow the student the opportunity to discuss with their mentors concerns that they may have and how effectively they are meeting the required competencies, outcomes or proficiencies in an attempt to enhance that placement as an effective learning environment. It will also provide an opportunity to give the student both positive and negative feedback as required.

However, Duffy (2004) found that mentors were 'failing to fail' some students who were not achieving in practice, thereby students were being signed off as being competent without appropriate justification. Some mentors would argue that it is much easier to sign to verify that a student has achieved, rather than becoming involved in providing statements or verbal evidence as part of an educational inquiry into the student's failure to achieve. It would therefore be useful for mentors to discuss any concerns that they may have about a student's progress with the individual's personal tutor or another significant educational link from the School of Nursing.

The success of practice placements in establishing their reputation and profile as an area that is conducive to learning is dependent on a number of factors and variables that involve both the placement staff and the students themselves. To be successful it is important to ensure that an effective partnership is established where the mentor supports, guides and advises the student throughout their healthcare experience. This would be enhanced if mentors viewed mentorship as a positive aspect of their role and as an opportunity to enhance their professional development.

Throughout this chapter the main focus was a number of variables that influence the effectiveness of the practice placements from the healthcare student's perspective.

Frequently asked questions

Mentors

Q. Why do some students evaluate their experience at the end of their placement in a negative manner but yet do not express any concerns whilst on placement?

A. Unfortunately, this is not an unusual situation. At the end of each placement, students may be asked to complete a 'student evaluation of placement' or some other feedback evaluation either online, if available, or as a paper exercise. This is an important feedback process that is used as part of a quality assurance mechanism. If you ask students why they wait until they leave before they offer any negative feedback, they say this is part of their basic 'survival' process. Some students will not criticize the placement in case there are any negative repercussions.

Q. What is the point in making an effort to ensure the student's experience is valuable for them in the practice setting, when they don't appear to appreciate the mentor's contributions?

A. This is a disappointing question but nevertheless one that is asked at mentor updates. In accordance with NMC domain five, it is the mentor's responsibility to ensure that they meet the stated outcomes, so the efforts given should be valued. It sometimes appears that students don't appreciate all the planning and preparation that mentors are involved in to ensure that their practice experience is the best that can be attained. Mentors have to balance this negative viewpoint with the more frequent positive one of gratitude that students make in their positive evaluations and face-to-face thanks during the final interview. Feedback can be a worthwhile learning experience for mentors as it helps them to remain aware of what students want from them.

Students

Q. Why do some staff agree to be a mentor when they obviously really don't want to take on that role?

A. Unfortunately, students do not always appreciate the diversity of a qualified nurse's role and responsibilities, despite the fact that this is emphasized by lecturers in the higher education institute. For some qualified staff, undertaking the role of a mentor is not welcomed as enthusiastically as it is by others, sometimes it may be viewed as a necessity to justify their professional banding or as a prerequisite for promotion. However, hopefully this applies to the minority of mentors.

(Continued)

(Continued)

Q. Why have some mentors forgotten what it is like being a student, having to work in placement and complete written assignments at the same time?

A. Sometimes this may be viewed as a rhetorical question because some mentors are undertaking further studies as part of their Lifelong Learning: Learning Beyond Registration Programme or to meet their PREP requirements (NMC, 2008c). However, it is a serious and thought-provoking question that students do pose and the answer is not an easy one, the answer appears to be a personal issue for the mentor themselves.

Chapter summary

This chapter has focused on the various issues that influence what makes a placement effective for healthcare students. Having completed the chapter, you have learned about:

- the contributory factors that make an 'effective' placement for healthcare students and the variables of the practice placement, mentorship and resources;
- a number of established 'checklists', these have been described and compared with that generated by discussions with student nurses;
- the need to maintain an interprofessional approach and how the general principles examined relate to various healthcare students;
- the need to ensure that the mentor's interest and their enthusiasm to reflect on their practice placement must be rejuvenated.

Further reading

Health Professions Council (HPC) (2008) *Your Duties as a Registrant: Standards of Conduct, Performance and Ethics*. London: HPC.

Royal College of Nursing (RCN) (2007b) *Guidance for Mentors of Nursing Students and Midwives: An RCN Toolkit*, 2nd edn. London: RCN.

Both documents contain useful and supportive information for mentors of healthcare students. They elaborate on the overall content examined throughout this chapter and both can be used as a valuable placement resource for both students and healthcare professionals.

7

The practice context in healthcare settings

David Kinnell

Nursing and Midwifery Council (2008a): Eight domains of mentorship Domain Six: Context of practice

Aim

Support learning within a context of practice that reflects healthcare and educational policies, managing change to ensure that particular professional needs are met within a learning environment that also supports practice development.

Outcomes

Stage 1: Nurses and Midwives

- Whilst enhancing their own practice and proficiency, a registered nurse or midwife act as a role model to others to enable them to learn their unique professional role.

Stage 2: Mentor

- Contribute to the development of an environment in which effective practice is fostered, implemented, evaluated and disseminated.
- Set and maintain professional boundaries that are sufficiently flexible for providing interprofessional care.
- Initiate and respond to practice developments to ensure safe and effective care is achieved and an effective learning environment is maintained.

Introduction

Throughout the NMC (2008a) developmental framework to support learning and assessment in practice, the eight domains all identify a specific focus that will help to guide and support mentors involved in the process of mentorship. These domains are generic and offer suggestions for all mentors of nursing, midwifery and healthcare students. This chapter will focus on domain six which relates to the context of practice. A number of themes are identified both in the aim and outcomes for both Stage One and Stage Two mentors, these have been amalgamated and will be explored under two main headings:

- Supporting learning within the context of practice.
- Responding to academic changes, in the practice setting.

Supporting learning within the context of practice

The overarching theme throughout this domain six capitalizes on the previous domain five whereby once an effective environment has been created, it then needs to be maintained and further enhanced. There is also a link between both Stage One and Stage Two mentors – the need to value and establish the importance of facilitation of learning and the process of assessment. It would therefore appear that domain six reaffirms the conceptual ideology of mentorship but then encourages a further exploration of the significance of those factors that may influence the success of dissemination and maintenance of safe and effective care within a healthcare environment.

Jones (2008a: 261) states: 'Supporting students to learn together *and* from each other, along with encouraging a sharing of their knowledge and know-how with others constitutes important experiential learning.' Reflecting on this statement, mentors supporting learning have to ensure that their knowledge and skills reflect the most recent amendments and adaptations to the process of mentorship. For both Stage One and Stage Two mentors, the effectiveness of enhancing learning is counteracted by their awareness of the process of assessment and interrelatedness of these two mentorship roles. Now complete Mentor Activity 7.1 before continuing with this chapter. This will encourage you to reflect on your own practice placement and ensure that your orientation programme for healthcare students remains as effective as you would like it to be.

MENTOR ACTIVITY 7.1

How do you welcome a healthcare student to your practice area?

Consider this question before continuing with this chapter.

In the practice context it is important to reflect on and evaluate the effectiveness of the welcoming process that the healthcare student undergoes as part of their orientation into your practice placement. Therefore, consider your responses to the Mentor Activity 7.1 as you read through the next section.

Welcoming the student to the practice placement

It is anticipated that the healthcare student will be met by their allocated mentor on the first day on placement. This will subsequently allow the mentor the opportunity to start the orientation process, explaining any specific security codes or processes, and introducing them to other members of the team, patients, clients, service users and their relatives, where appropriate. In some practice placements there are specific issues that need to be discussed as part of that orientation process:

- Medical Emergency Procedure (cardiac arrest alert call telephone number);
- location of emergency equipment;
- fire exits and procedure in case of an emergency;
- moving and handling equipment use and location;
- staff communication boards/books, general and specific.

Each student usually has a series of three interviews throughout the duration of their placement depending on the time duration. The following is an example of how that tripartite approach to practice-based interviews could be orchestrated.

The preliminary interview

Each student nurse will arrive with their specific documentation, associated with their specific training programme and this needs to be completed accordingly. Some students will need to have a preliminary or initial interview, on the first day or as soon as possible thereafter. This will allow the mentor and student time to discuss the specific practice-based learning needs. Student nurses will have to achieve their Outcomes for Entry to Branch or Achievement of

Standards of Proficiency for Entry to the NMC Professional Register, these later requirements are related to years two and three of their selected Branch Programme (NMC, 2004c). These may vary according to specific programmes, so you will need to ascertain with the student the requirements that they have to attain. Whatever the training programme (extended – part-time; diploma; degree; shortened post-graduate or masters), students do need the mentor's assistance in helping and guiding them to achieve their requirements. The NMC (2008a) recommend that students spend at least 40% of their practice placement with a mentor, preferably their own identified mentor.

The preliminary interview will allow the student to identify any specific learning needs that they may have and give the mentor the chance to discuss how they will be achieved. The student may have some existing placement outcomes or proficiencies to achieve from their previous placement that can be highlighted and discussed. It is hoped that the mentor will assist the student to compile an action plan based on what they hope to achieve and the mechanism of achieving those requirements.

The student nurse may have specific academic assessments to complete whilst on placement, including written assignments, worksheet activities and practical preparations for their OSCEs (Objective Structured/Simulation Clinical Examinations) as indicated by the Nursing and Midwifery Council (2006a; 2008a). Murray et al. (2008) emphasize how significant simulation has become within today's educational climate. Also, the academic requirements can be discussed with the mentor and guidance given on how they can be achieved, based on an individualistic approach. The student could highlight any specific practice-based weaknesses that they may have and wish to further develop. This interview provides an opportunity to identify the student's individual needs in respect of achieving the Essential Skills Clusters assessments (NMC, 2007a) and to plan how the placement experience will help to achieve those needs.

It is anticipated that students will have a follow-up interview, the intermediate interview and then, a final interview (RCN, 2004). It may be appropriate to set dates and times of these two interviews, so that the mentor and student are aware of what will happen over the next few weeks and give a specific date to work towards. The mentor and student can discuss how they will collect the evidence to meet the placement outcomes or proficiencies. This will provide the student with a structured, self-directed approach to utilizing their time most effectively.

The intermediate interview

Approximately half-way through the placement, it is advisable for the mentor to have a discussion with their student to review the progress made. This interaction will allow the opportunity to ascertain how successful the student has been in establishing effective working relationships so far in the practice placement and any problems encountered. For some higher education institutes, this may be viewed as the most important interview because it will allow the mentor to discuss with the student:

- how well the student feels that they are developing their knowledge and practice-based skills;
- which outcomes or proficiencies have been achieved, and how many more need to be attained;
- the type and quality of evidence the student is producing to ensure that they are meeting the NMC (2004a: 34);
- which insight visits to other significant healthcare settings the student has attended, and what other potential areas are included in the itinerary list that they could visit that would enhance their learning.

However, the most important aspect of this interview is to use the experience in order to highlight to the student any areas of concern. If the mentor is concerned about any of the following:

- communication and interpersonal skills;
- standard of nursing care delivery and hence development of practice-based competencies and skills;
- safety of patients, clients or the student involving issues such as moving and handling, infection control, and maintenance of a safe environment;
- professional behaviour, for example, attendance, personal appearance, punctuality, time keeping;
- establishing effective working relationships within the interprofessional team and if there are any conflicts, how they are being managed and resolved.

These will all contribute to the placement profile and its effectiveness as an area for effective learning.

It is important therefore to review the preliminary interview, reiterate what was intended and to what extent those expectations are being met. If an action plan was initiated, it would be appropriate to review its content and amend it according to the discourse generated at this meeting. Any areas of weakness need to be identified and the mentor must discuss ways of helping the student to achieve the deficits. A time limit needs to be established in order to assist the student to work towards achieving those weaknesses.

Unfortunately, this is one of the roles that some mentors feel uncomfortable having to undertake but nevertheless feedback is necessary. It is advisable that mentors start on a positive note, emphasizing the overall progress made so far, before introducing the negative areas of concern. This can be turned into a positive, supportive interaction if the action plan is reviewed, and amended so that any advice on how to achieve the areas of concern are clearly stated and agreed. On short or insight placements, it may not be possible to undertake this interview.

The final interview

During the last week of placement it is necessary to undertake the final interview, and complete the student's documentation. Throughout the practice placement, the process of continuous assessment will ensure that all the required competencies, outcomes or proficiencies have been achieved. It is advisable that mentors avoid episodic assessments whereby they assess the student's achievements only in the last week because this does not provide the opportunity to highlight areas of weakness that could be turned into a positive development. If these are identified during the placement, then they can be improved in the last few weeks in placement and, hence, ensure that the student feels that they have enjoyed the practice-based experience and have been supported throughout. The student can then finish the placement with the documentation complete, and any areas for future development identified ready for the next placement – this is seen as a positive developmental feedback and gives the mentor a positive sense of accomplishment.

Unfortunately, in some instances, the mentors do not complete the documentation in time so the student has to leave the practice placement not knowing how successful they have been. An interview implies that there has been some interaction between two people. For a number of reasons, the mentor does not complete the Assessment of Practice Record which causes distress to the student because they have to arrange to return and collect their completed document at a later date. Alternatively some mentors will return the documentation by internal mail to the School of Nursing, not allowing the student the chance to discuss it in the final interview. This situation is made worse if the mentor states that the student has failed to achieve some of the competencies, outcomes or proficiencies due to insufficient evidence, or poor unsafe practice, thus, they have subsequently been denied the opportunity to discuss that final decision. This is an inappropriate approach to mentorship and one that must be avoided.

However, this situation will become a thing of the past because of the Ongoing Achievement Record (Continuity of Practice Assessment Record) which has been used by pre-registration students since September 2007 (NMC, 2006a). Mentorship is time-consuming, challenging but nevertheless extremely rewarding, providing the process is adhered to. Undertaking the series of three interviews in the practice context is useful for the student but also helps the mentors with the process of assessment and interpretation.

Therefore, mentors need to familiarize themselves with the process of assessment and accountability and how changes are made in accordance with NMC recommendations. There are a number of inherent challenges of assessment and these need to be considered in order to facilitate the success of the process, and distinguish between a realistic and an unrealistic outcome. The emphasis on accountability now requires mentors to fully appreciate their importance within the assessment process, within the practice context. Unfortunately, as stated by Duffy and Hardicre (2007a) some mentors do not realize the significance of this accountability and subsequently are 'failing to fail' students. The importance of mentors assessing students is to ensure that they maintain safety and 'protect the public' (NMC, 2008a).

The NMC (2004c) established the *Standards of Proficiency for Pre-registration Nursing Education* and thus introduced a framework of assessing the achievement of skills within the practice setting. These are based on four domains (see Box 7.1).

Box 7.1   Standards of proficiency domains

Domain One – Professional and Ethical Practice
Domain Two – Care Delivery
Domain Three – Care Management
Domain Four – Personal and Professional Development

(NMC, 2004c)

They are subsequently identified as:

- Outcomes for Entry to Branch: Common Foundation Programme;
- Standards of Proficiency for Entry to the NMC Professional Register.

These are presented in the documentation that student nurses bring with them to the practice area, when they work with their mentor, in order to achieve sufficient evidence that they have met the stated criteria. This documentation, although the design may differ in each higher education institute, should constitute an effective assessment tool that will ensure parity for all students, as they all have the same outcomes or proficiencies to achieve.

TABLE 7.1   *Comparison of different Pre-registration Training Programmes*

Three-year Pre-registration Training Programme A	Training Programme B
0–6 months = Helper or novice status	0–6 months = Practice Level One
6–18 months = Supervised Participant	6–12 months = Practice Level Two
18–30 months = Participant	12–24 months = Practice Level Three
30–36 months = Assistant to First Level Nurse	24–36 months = Practice Level Four

Source: (Bondy, 1983).

A number of assessment tools are used and the expectations required by each student nurse according to their level of training, needs to be clearly explained to all mentors involved in supporting learning within the team. It is hoped that this will allow for an ipsative approach to assessment whereby the student's progress can be ascertained by comparing their level at the start of the placement and that achieved at the end. Some Stage One mentors working alongside and observing the Stage Two mentor will be able to gain an awareness of how the process is executed before they themselves undertake a Nursing and Midwifery Council Approved Mentor Preparation Training Programme. At each stage of the student nurse's training the expectations associated with that level should be clearly defined (Table 7.1).

Different higher education institutes will have their own adaptation to this framework so the mentor must familiarize themselves with their local guidelines.

Irrespective of the training programme, the specific indicators or descriptors for each level must be defined so that the mentor can discuss their expectations of the student nurse during their preliminary/initial interview, as part of the orientation programme. This will provide the opportunity for the student nurse to identify their specific learning expectations and needs so that the mentor can specify those that are realistically achievable. Stage One mentors can contribute to supporting learning for students as directed by the NMC (2008b: 6): 'You must make sure that everyone that you are responsible for is supervised and supported' and 'You must keep your knowledge and skills up to date throughout your working life. You must take part in appropriate learning and practice activities that maintain and develop your competence and performance' (ibid.: 7).

As a supportive team, mentors work in partnership with the student to help support and guide the student nurse throughout their practice placement. However, in reality, this contribution is not an equal partnership and some student nurses, for whatever reasons, fail to show an interest in their own development which causes a sensitive situation within the practice team who are trying to support that student's learning. This emphasizes the relevance of accountability as part of the mentor's approach to effective mentorship. Duffy (2004) identified that some mentors actually 'failed to fail' students for a number of potential reasons which had implications for the student nurse and for other future mentors. Accountability is juxtaposed alongside honesty and having the confidence to state that the student is not achieving the level expected whilst in the practice setting. If the mentor has any justifiable concerns regarding a student's behaviour, development or progress they should contact someone significant either academic or practice link, to discuss these issues (NMC, 2009).

Duffy and Hardicre (2007b) highlight the importance of *supporting failing students in practice* and as found in Duffy's (2004) research, problems do need to be confronted, explored and discussed although the experience can be extremely emotive. Mentors either have intuitive knowledge that there are intra-personal issues or as displayed by the healthcare student's overt behaviour, there may be 'attitude problems' that are complex and not always objectively managed.

Duffy and Hardicre (2007b: 28) offer a checklist of 'Practical advice for mentors' in order to provide feedback to the healthcare student:

- Arrange for all meetings with students to be held in a private area.
- Ensure students have prior notification of the meeting.
- Ensure there will be no interruptions, such as phone calls.
- Put plenty of time aside for the meeting.

Mentors can then explore how to deal with the student. This is a realistic plan of action that could be implemented in order to enhance the effectiveness of giving constructive negative feedback to the healthcare student in a positive manner.

However, after discussing this issue with third-year students (in their last six months of training), their reflective discourse appears to be entrenched in negative descriptions of their unfortunate experiences of mentorship mismanagement.

Responding to academic changes in the practice setting

Change is an important perspective if the National Health Service is to continually develop to meet contemporary health care needs. Iles and Sutherland (2001) emphasize that implementing an aspect of change into the NHS may incur challenges from the following:

- changing pressures in the environment;
- changing technologies available;
- complex organizations in which individuals and teams are interdependent.

Tomey (2004) and Marquis and Huston (2006) state that the process of change can be influenced by a number of cultural differences: values and norms; beliefs and attitudes; mental processes and learning styles. These also may have an impact on the success of implementing change. Unfortunately, mentors have to juggle change management both in the context of practice as well as in the academic support of healthcare students.

One of the most recent changes in nurse education that will have a direct impact on mentors is the introduction of the Essential Skills Clusters for Pre-registration Nursing programmes that were introduced by the NMC (2007a; 2007b). The Essential Skills Clusters are intended to complement the NMC (2004c) Nursing Standards and they must be introduced into all new Pre-registration Nurse Training Programmes from September 2008. According to the NMC (2007a: 1):

> The ESCs have been developed as an outcome of the Review of fitness for practice at the point of registration; they aim to provide clarity of expectation for the public and profession alike and seek to address some of the concerns about skill deficits arising from the Review.

The essential skills clusters

The Essential Skills Clusters for Nursing and Midwifery are therefore a set of national skills statements that are intended to support the existing NMC (2004c) outcomes for entry to the branch, and the proficiencies for entry to the register, they are not a substitute for them. The skills have been identified as those that are deemed essential rather than trying to incorporate all skills that relate to specific aspects of practice. The ESCs that have been introduced into nursing in 2008 focus on five different aspects and relate to 42 statements identifying what the patient/client can trust a newly registered nurse to do (see Box 7.2).

Box 7.2   The Essential Skills Clusters

- Care, Compassion and Communication (8 statements)
- Organizational aspects of care (12 statements)
- Infection prevention and control (6 statements)
- Nutrition and fluid maintenance (6 statements)
- Medicines management (10 statements)

(NMC 2007a, 2007b)

The NMC emphasizes that the Essential Skills Clusters identify skills that:

- are under broad headings fundamental to best practice;
- relate to all nursing fields of practice;
- reflect patient expectation of new qualifiers in specific areas;
- complement existing NMC outcomes and proficiencies;
- are required to be incorporated within all pre-registration nursing programmes;
- require specific testing;
- require to be demonstrated before entry to the branch programme and prior to registration;
- will be subject to ongoing monitoring and review. (NMC, 2007a: 2)

To facilitate the introduction of the Essential Skills Clusters, the NMC have produced three separate documents, Annexes One, Two and Three, that provide an explanation of the rationale and historical background, a checklist of the 42 statements and a mapping document related to the Nursing Standards (NMC, 2004c). In Annexe Two, the statements are presented and link to other significant documents including:

- Outcomes and proficiencies within the *Standards of Proficiency for Pre-registration Nursing Education* (NMC, 2004c);
- the Code of Professional Conduct: Standards for Conduct, Performance and Ethics (NMC, 2004b).

The NMC specifies the 'Items requiring numerical assessment' and 'Items requiring specific assessment' (NMC, 2007a). In Annexe Two are the summative health-related numerical assessments within the ESCs that require baseline assessment and calculations associated with:

- medicines
- nutrition
- fluids
- other areas requiring the use of numbers relevant to the context of practice.

Schools of Nursing and Midwifery within higher education institutes have been involved throughout 2008 in the planning and decision-making process to ascertain the most effective ways of assessing the Essential Skills Clusters and what stages throughout the student's Training Programme these skills will be assessed and by whom. The 42 statements follow the same format as the example shown and act as guidelines for mentors to help them appreciate the importance of their role within this summative process.

Throughout mentor preparation programmes and mentor updates, the Essential Skills Clusters and the specific assessment tools that mentors will be using have been a topic of discussion. However, since all pre-registration student nurses from September 2008 will be assessed based on these skills, it is important that all mentors contact their academic links to ensure that they are aware of the changes that have been implemented.

The first cohorts have already worked in the practice placement and mentors have already gained their first experience of assessing these practice-based Essential Skills Clusters assessments. In some placements, students have achieved all those required for the Common Foundation Programmes, some have achieved none, whilst others constitute a variety of achievements. What is extremely positive feedback from the mentors is the recognition and established value of their credibility in undertaking these summative assessments in practice.

There are a number of assessments to be undertaken in the Common Foundation Programme and others specific to the Branch Programme. Mentors have been introduced to the overall concept and have now gained their first experience, this will continue with support from the academic educational link as and when required.

An example of one of the 42 statements can be found in Box 7.3. Mentors must now accept more responsibility for these summative assessments of students in the practice placement throughout the Common Foundation Programme. An example of their assessment responsibility includes:

- Monitors Height, Weight and Body Mass Index
- Monitors and records Fluid Balance
- Monitors and records Dietary Intake.

Box 7.3   Trusting a newly qualified registered nurse

1. Patients/clients can trust a newly registered nurse to do the following: Provide care based on the highest standards, knowledge and competence.

For entry to branch

- Demonstrates the underpinning values of the *NMC Code of Professional Conduct: Standards for Conduct, Performance and Ethics*.
- Works within limitations of the role and recognizes own level of competence.
- Promotes a professional image.
- Shows respect for others.
- Is able to engage patients/clients and build caring professional relationships.
- Forms appropriate and constructive professional relationships with families and other carers.
- Uses professional support structures to learn from experience and make appropriate adjustments.

For entry to the register

- Demonstrates clinical confidence through sound knowledge, skills and understanding relevant to Branch.
- Is self-aware and self-confident, knows own limitations and is able to take appropriate action.
- Acts a role model in promoting a professional image.
- Acts a role model in developing trusting relationships, within professional boundaries.
- Recognizes and acts to overcome barriers in developing effective relationships with patients/clients.
- Initiates, maintains and closes professional relationships with patients/clients and carers.
- Uses professional support structures to develop self-awareness, challenge own prejudices and enable professional; relationships, so that care is delivered without compromise.

(NMC, 2007b, Annexe 2 to NMC Circular 07/2007)

Care, compassion and communication

The higher education institutes remain responsible for assessing vital body sign assessment (temperature, pulse and respiratory rate, as well as blood pressure measurement) = these can both be assessed in a summative OSCE format; whereas Aseptic Technique can be assessed using a simulation approach. Higher education institutes will devise their own assessment strategies of how these assessments will fulfil the NMC (2007a) requirements, those identified are an example.

When the student enters their chosen branch, the assessments will continue, the mentors will, according to the speciality, assess the students undertaking the following:

- Nutritional Assessment
- Hydration/Dehydration Assessment
- Enteral Feeding (Branch specific)
- Intravenous Fluid (Branch specific)
- Medicine Administration for an individual or small group.

These are practice-based assessments and the mentor will be provided with a criterion–specific assessment tool. These summative assessments only have to be passed once although the student will also be expected to continue developing their other practical skills. The student can practise and have as much formative experience as they feel they need but they will only be allowed two summative attempts in the practice placement. There will be variations of documentation and assessment criteria according to the individual Higher Education Institutes. As a mentor you need to familiarize yourself with local assessment strategies. The final assessment will be a Patient Group Directions – this could be a classroom-based assessment.

The implementation of the Essential Skills Clusters will have a significant impact on the mentor's role. In the past few years students have continually criticized the validity and reliability of the OSCEs, particularly as they are undertaken in the classroom setting, with a lecturer enacting the role of the patient. This situation was embarrassing for them and they felt the assessment was 'false'. However, the Essential Skills Clusters will now incorporate various assessment strategies that add an extra dimension to the mentor's ever evolving role but one which hopefully will be more satisfying and fulfilling for the mentor.

Equality and diversity in contemporary healthcare

Another important aspect of change that contributes to the development of an effective practice environment is a positive commitment to establish equality and diversity. This is a growing awareness of the individuality of healthcare students whilst the mentors are assessing them in the practice placement. They constitute an important awareness of how individual students actually learn in the practice placement.

Now complete Mentor Activity 7.2, and reflect of your views before continuing with this chapter.

MENTOR ACTIVITY 7.2

What factors do you think influence the importance of equality and diversity within your healthcare environment?

Reflect on your answer before continuing to read this chapter.

The NMC (2006a) emphasized the importance of disability equality training for mentors, and these have been reaffirmed in 2008. The NMC equality and diversity schemes implemented in 2007/2008 are, 'concerned with promoting equality of opportunity on the grounds of race, gender, and disability, and treating individuals with fairness, respect and understanding' (NMC, 2008a: 5). They subsequently highlight the importance of individuality and the need to appreciate that all healthcare students may have different needs and preferences that must be considered when assessing their learning styles and skills acquisition. This may influence the success of achieving the practice-based outcomes or proficiencies (NMC, 2004c), whilst in the healthcare environment. Mentors must be aware and respect the student's individuality, so review your answer to Mentor Activity 7.2.

There are three influential legislative documents that advocate the importance of valuing the rights of healthcare students who have a disability (see Box 7.4).

Box 7.4   Disability Discrimination Acts

- The Disability Discrimination Act (Parliament, 1995)
- The Disability Discrimination Act (Parliament, 2005)
- The Special Educational Needs and Disability Act (Parliament, 2001)

These Acts contain important recommendations that have an impact both in the educational and healthcare practice settings. It is therefore the mentor's responsibility to ensure that they are aware of these recommendations so that in the practice context they can support the student to ensure that they are involved in delivering safe and effective care. Now complete Mentor Activity 7.3.

MENTOR ACTIVITY 7.3

What are some of the main recommendations within these three Disability Acts?

Reflect on your response before continuing.

The Disability Discrimination Act (Parliament, 1995)

This was the first significant document that highlighted that it was no longer acceptable to discriminate against disabled people in employment and they should also have access to good services. The main emphasis was the right to expect reasonable adjustments and the responsibility of employers to consider how they supported people (service users and staff) with disabilities. The Health Professions Council (2007g) highlight that the Disability Discrimination Act (1995) is a significant piece of legislation that aims to protect the individual with a disability. They state: 'Education providers have responsibilities to their students and applicants to make sure that they are treated fairly' and 'Employers have a duty to their employees and to applicants' (HPC, 2007g: 2).

Special Education Needs and Disability Act (Parliament, 2001)

This Act was introduced in order to place responsibilities on educational institutions to ensure that students with disabilities were no longer treated differently, unfavourably, and therefore the educational institutions had to implement reasonable adjustments as deemed necessary. These recommended changes included:

- making changes to policies and practices;
- changing course requirements or work placements;
- altering the physical features of a building;
- providing interpreters or other support workers;
- delivering courses in alternative ways;
- providing learning materials in other formats (RCN, 2007b).

The Disability Discrimination Act (Parliament, 2005)

This Act was an updated version of the one previously introduced a decade earlier but with the additional introduction of the requirements for all public authorities to promote disability equality, to provide disability equality schemes, to monitor and publish progress reports. Subsequently, 'all public authorities were required to produce a *disability equality scheme* by December 2006' according to the RCN (2007b: 19). Reflect on your existing knowledge and understanding by completing Mentor Activity 7.4.

MENTOR ACTIVITY 7.4

What is a disability?

Reflect on your response before continuing.

What is meant by disability?

There are two approaches that emphasize the importance of understanding 'what is disability?'

1   *Medical model of disability* – this is related to overt impairment and loss of function.
2   *Social model of disability* – refers to environmental, societal and attitudinal barriers that are themselves disabling for the individual.

However, mentors need to appreciate that students have adapted to their health problems and impairments and hence do not perceive themselves as significantly disabled. Alternatively, there may be a self-fulfilling prophecy whereby if the student declares that they have a disability, they may feel that they will be labelled and suffer the associated stigma given to them by healthcare staff (HPC, 2005). In order to support a student, the mentor therefore needs to be non-judgemental, sensitive, and to respect the student with non-conditional positive regard.

The RCN (2007b: 18) highlights that some of the more common impairments and disabilities that students may have include:

- dyslexia and/or dyscalculia;
- epilepsy;
- hearing or visual impairment;
- progressive medical conditions;
- mental health conditions;
- physical disability and/or restricted mobility.

Dyslexia

The word 'dyslexia' originates from the Greek language and means 'difficulty with words'. It is, 'a specific learning difficulty which mainly affects the development of literacy and language related skills' (British Dyslexia Association, 2007). According to Turkington and Harris (2006), the incidence of dyslexia is estimated to occur in approximately 8 per cent of the population. Although dyslexia may be viewed as problematic there are complementary compensations with the individual developing strengths in abilities such as creativity or physical co-ordination. Mentors must realize and appreciate that each student with dyslexia can suffer varying degrees from mild to severe disruptions in their learning capacity.

The problems with reading reported by dyslexics are associated with intelligence or motivation. In contrast, people with dyslexia often have unusual talents related to areas that require visual, spatial and motor skills. The fundamental differentiation with dyslexia is relative to how the brain processes information whilst the person is reading. Although dyslexia is a permanent feature, with appropriate guidance and support, individuals may largely overcome and deal with their reading difficulties, (ibid.). Mentors must appreciate that some students are unaware of their dyslexia before commencing their nursing or midwifery training.

The RCN (2007b) presents a checklist for mentors so that they understand how dyslexia may affect the student, this includes:

- erratic spelling;
- misreading;
- poor handwriting;
- poor memory retention;
- difficulty in organizing work;
- poor time management;
- short concentration span;
- confusion between right and left.

The British Dyslexia Association (2007) also includes the following:

- reading hesitantly;
- difficulty with sequences, e.g. getting dates in order;
- difficulty organizing thoughts clearly.

This is an extremely useful, concise summary which clearly identifies how dyslexia may impact on the healthcare student's cognitive functioning.

Dyscalculia

This is a disability that concerns mentors because of the potential of drug errors whilst undertaking drug calculations. Turkington and Harris (2006) identify that this is a learning disability associated with mathematics. The individual may have difficulty understanding the concept of simple numbers, lack an intuitive grasp of numbers, and have problems learning number facts and procedures. Hence, there is a problem with learning or applying mathematical concepts, functions and procedures. This is further complicated because although they may be able to produce the desired arithmetical answer or use a correct method, they may do this in a mechanistic manner rather than in a deductive confident approach.

How can mentors support a student with dyslexia in the practice setting?

There are a number of reasonable adjustments that can be considered in order to support healthcare students in practice providing the practice placement is notified before the student arrives. However, some students may not want to advertise their disability until they actually arrive on placement and this is revealed as part of the initial/preliminary interview. The RCN (2007b: 21) offers a really useful list of suggestions of how mentors can support their healthcare students:

- Provide the student with a glossary of terms or medical jargon before they start the placement – this is often incorporated in a welcoming, orientation or information pack.
- Ask the student what their typical difficulties are and how they 'normally cope', and how you can support them.
- Limit written work in groups to avoid embarrassment and feelings of inadequacy.
- Ask questions clearly and concisely.
- Give instructions in sequences, and allow pauses when communicating.
- Offer demonstrations and provide clear instructions and expectations and be aware of information overload.
- When contributing to patient records, offer the student a supervised run on practice documentation before allowing entries on a legal document.
- Ensure calculations are taken independently; allow time, and always double check.

- Ask the student to write out the calculation, so you can identify the type or stage of any error. The RCN (2007b: 22) states, 'Impairment does not mean incapacity. With appropriate support, students with disabilities can work well in clinical as well as academic settings and can add value to clinical practice from their personal experiences.' Unfortunately, there is a difference between idealism and reality, read Case study 7.1, for a real experience of mentorship within contemporary healthcare.

CASE STUDY 7.1

A mentor approached a student nurse and asked her what was wrong with her. The mentor stated, 'I explained this to you yesterday, why do I have to explain this again?' The student nurse replied stating that she wanted to make sure that she was doing the right thing.

The mentor's response was, 'Unless you're "thick", I shouldn't have to explain things twice.'

The student nurse was upset by what the mentor had said, her voice intonation and the condescending manner in which she spoke. She subsequently explained to her mentor that she had dyslexia.

The mentor's reply was, 'Maybe you're in the wrong job.'

This was a distressing conversation for the student who was trying to be honest with her mentor but the reciprocal response was negative and discriminatory.

How could this experience have been more positive for both those involved?

In contrast, the Health Professions Council (2005) clearly explores the impact of disability equality in their document *A Disabled Person's Guide to Becoming a Health Professional: Consultative Document*, in which they offer reassurance that disabled people who previously would not have considered a career as a health care professional may make an informed decision about their career pathway. In this document, they differentiate, 'between being *registered* as a health professional and being *employed* as a health professional' (HPC, 2005: 14). The role of the HPC is to engage in the registration of healthcare professionals and clearly not to deal with matters associated with the employment of the individual. Furthermore, the health professional should not perceive registration as a guarantee of employment.

All healthcare professional registrants must practise within their identified 'scope of practice' as a conditional component of gaining their registration. 'A health professional's scope of practice is the area or areas of their profession in which they have the knowledge, skills and experience to practise safely and effectively' (HPC, 2005: 19). They subsequently have to ensure that they do not endanger themselves or the public if there is a change in their personal circumstances as a result of a disability or a health issue.

For some registrants, as part of their registration, they have a responsibility to ensure that the HPC standards are adhered to. However, sometimes the employer has responsibilities under the Disability Discrimination Act (2005). In contrast, now read Case study 7.2 to illustrate how the two different responsibilities can work together to ensure that the public, as well as the disabled person, are protected. There is a marked contrast of experience between Case study 7.2 and Case study 7.1.

CASE STUDY 7.2

An occupational therapist with multiple sclerosis became ill again. He became concerned about his ability to perform certain aspects of his job safely and effectively.

He discussed his condition with his employer, and together they agreed various changes to the way that he worked. For example, he would be accompanied on home visits by an assistant. The assistant would also perform any manual handling that was needed. The employer and employee would investigate 'Access to Work' which could provide funding needed for these adjustments.

The employer agreed that the support would be ongoing, and also that they would continue to meet regularly, to make sure that the adjustments made could be reviewed and changed if necessary. The employee agreed to update his employer on any further changes to his condition.

(Health Professions Council, 2007g: 8)

How could you as a mentor respond to a situation like this?

From the individual person's perspective the experience in both case studies varied. Jones (2008a: 262) highlights this difference and states:

> Insensitive viewpoints about vulnerable groups of learners have not necessarily been moderated in recent years by educational reforms. Therefore, possibly in systematic ways, unhelpful and undetected attitudes to those finding difficulties in achieving can be passed on throughout educational structures, alongside clinical settings.

Student Support Services are committed to providing appropriately accessible services and supporting students in order to facilitate the successful completion of their course, their learning and their training as independently as possible. The range of support services available may include:

- Academic Support, including Dyslexia Support and Disability Support Teams.
- Student Services Centre that provides assessments for students who have applied for Disabled Students' Allowance.
- Academic Support also incorporates study support which offers help and guidance with academic writing skills and time management.
- Disability Liaison Officers (DLO).
- Disability Policy Advisory Unit (DPAU) which ensures that the recommendations in the Special Educational Needs and Disability Act (2001) and the Disability Discrimination Act (2005) are adhered to.

- Advisory Group on Disability (AGD).
- Students' Union – Students with Disabilities Association.

Higher education institutes may also provide guidance on 'Disability Equality Schemes' in which the Scheme capitalizes on both the Disability Discrimination Acts of 1995 and 2005, responding to public authorities, requirements to have regard to the need to do the following:

- Eliminate unlawful discrimination.
- Eliminate unlawful harassment.
- Eliminate unlawful victimization.
- Promote equality of opportunity between disabled persons' circumstances, even where that involves treating disabled persons more favourably than other persons.
- Promote positive attitudes towards disabled people.
- Encourage greater participation by disabled people in the life of the University and in public life more generally. (University of Nottingham, 2006: 4)

Despite these supportive strategies there still may be challenges in the practice setting for healthcare students. Now read Case study 7.3 for a very disturbing experience involving a student when she asked, 'Why did the staff treat me like this?' This was a negative experience that could have been avoided if the staff members had ensured that they understood the extent of this student's problem. The NMC (2008a) has recommended that disability equality training should be accessible to all mentors.

Unfortunately, as part of the five-day theory content within the new ten-day programme (NMC, 2008a) for Stage Two mentor training, it is difficult to explore disability equality effectively. So instead of training, mentors merely gain an awareness, insight or update on how to support students with a disability rather than an in-depth disability training. This may vary in individual higher education institutes. Mentors do need to reflect therefore on their own understanding and seek appropriate guidance from those trained appropriately, such as a Disability Liaison Officer or equivalent.

CASE STUDY 7.3

A student was on a placement and during the first week she confided in her mentor that she had dyslexia because she wanted to be open and hoped that in a reciprocal manner, the mentor would respect her individuality. The mentor proceeded to discuss with her colleagues that the student had dyslexia.

One day whilst working in the placement, the student walked into the Staff Room where she realized that the staff were sniggering and laughing, unsure why, she shrugged it off and continued to make herself a drink.

(Continued)

(Continued)

Some of the staff members then picked up a magazine and said to each other in an apparent derogatory manner:

'What does that say?'
'What does that mean?'

They then continued to snigger and laugh. The student was excluded from any conversation and ignored during the break. The student was made to feel uncomfortable and an outsider.

She later asked her mentor what the topic of the joke was because she felt that it had been directed at her and the fact that she had dyslexia. The mentor was evasive, did not reassure the student and this subsequently was the start of an uncomfortable and sensitive mentorship experience for this student.

What can you learn from this situation?

This situation could be viewed in different ways. The student may have misinterpreted the situation and hence it was not as insensitive as it appears. However, this is an interesting case study for mentors to consider and reflect on how they would avoid such an interaction.

Frequently asked questions

Mentors

Q. How can I support a student who has a disability without making them feel labelled or stigmatized? I want to help them but I don't want to embarrass them.

A. Each healthcare student is an individual and expects to be treated the same as any other student. If they have a disability, it could be assumed that they have adapted and have learnt to cope within the limitations that they may have. What is expected is that the student will discuss with their mentors their expectations and to what extent the mentor can be supportive. However, in the practice context, the student, like any others, is there to develop their knowledge, skills and attitudes to help them in preparation to becoming a healthcare professional. You need to identify the Student Support Services that are available for your healthcare students, and contact the supportive Disability Liaison Officer for further guidance.

Q. Are there any specific learning resources that we can obtain for practice to help the student with a disability maximize their learning within our ward environment?

A. This is a question that you could discuss with the student during their initial/preliminary interview. The RCN (2007b: 21) states that you could:

- provide the student with a glossary of terms before the placement starts;
- ask the student if they prefer receiving material on coloured paper.

Try and explore the more effective individualized way of supporting the healthcare student and this will hopefully enhance future learning when mentoring other students with a disability.

Students

Q. Whilst on a recent placement, I took a coloured acetate, which helps me to read and asked if I could leave it on the Nurses' Station. The mentor agreed but asked me to get permission from the manager who subsequently agreed that this would not be a problem. I hung the acetate in a folder, in a discreet place but when I returned the next day, it had been destroyed. This made my learning difficult and reduced my ability to function for the rest of that day – it was like having my glasses ripped off my face. The coloured acetate helps me to function safely and competently, so why was it destroyed?

A. The Disability Discrimination Act (1995) advocates the importance of making 'reasonable adjustments'. The RCN (2007b) emphasizes that a coloured acetate or overlay may help the student to function more effectively in the practice setting. So why was this student's 'minimal' reasonable adjustment contravened in accordance with the statutory recommendations, within the 'caring' profession of nursing?

Q. Whilst on placement I asked my mentor what action the drug frusemide had, why was it given intravenously, what was it mixed with and why? The time was appropriate, my mentor was not too busy, so it seemed a convenient time to ask the questions. I am trying to increase my understanding of drugs, their uses, ways of administration and their basic actions, so I didn't think I was being unreasonable. My mentor was not helpful, yes, she abruptly stated that frusemide reduces excess fluid and it is mixed with … However, because I have dyslexia I need things explaining a little slower, in order to be more effective. How much training do mentors get regarding supporting healthcare students with dyslexia?

(Continued)

(Continued)

A. The Nursing and Midwifery Council in 2006 and more recently 2008, advocates the importance of including disability equality training within Mentor Preparation Programmes. Related to equality and diversity, the NMC (2008a: 5) states that mentors should be 'treating individuals with fairness, respect and understanding … recognising that students have many different learning needs and preferences'.

Chapter summary

This chapter has explored the practice context examining both supporting learning and the importance of managing change. Having completed this chapter you have learned about:

- the effective process of welcoming a student into the practice placement in order to initiate the process of mentorship;
- the importance of the tripartite approach to student interviews within the continuous assessment process;
- what the Essential Skills Clusters for Pre-registration Nursing Programmes are and how they will be incorporated into mentorship;
- the importance of equality and diversity within contemporary healthcare and how this may have an impact on students;
- the need for disability equality training to be introduced within Mentor Preparation Programmes.

Further reading

Royal College of Nursing (2007b) *Guidance for Mentors of Nursing Students and Midwives: An RCN Toolkit,* 2nd edn. London: RCN.

Chapter 7 deals with 'students with disabilities' and is an effective concise overview of disability training for mentors.

Health Professions Council (2007g) *A Guide for Prospective Registrants and Admissions Staff: A Disabled Person's Guide to Becoming a Health Professional.* London: HPC.

This is a really useful document that explores the importance of disability awareness and how it can influence the allied professions who are seeking training and employment. This provides an extremely useful collection of case studies that involve a number of healthcare professionals who have a disability.

8

Evidence-based practice and mentorship

David Kinnell

Nursing and Midwifery Council (2008a): Eight domains of mentorship
Domain Seven: Evidence-based practice

Aim

Apply evidence-based practice to their own work and contribute to the further development of such knowledge and practice evidence base.

Outcomes

Stage 1: Nurses and Midwives

- Further develop their evidence base for practice to support their own personal and professional development and to contribute to the development of others.

Stage 2: Mentor

- Identify and apply research and evidence-based practice to their area of practice.
- Contribute to strategies to increase or review the evidence base used to support practice.
- Support students in applying an evidence base to their own practice.

Introduction

The importance of evidence-based practice was originally identified in the 1970s but it wasn't until the 1990s that this approach to nursing was given the acknowledgement that it deserved. The Department of Health (DH) (1991) emphasized why research and development was an essential component in the delivery of effective healthcare. Therefore, in the subsequent document *Research for Health*, the Department of Health (1991) clarified that research should, 'become an integral part of health care and that practitioners would find it necessary, and indeed natural, to base their daily decisions on research evidence' (Foundation of Nursing Studies, 2001: 4). The government and healthcare professionals supported the need for an evidence-based health service. This was documented in a series of reports by the Department of Health (1989, 1996a, 1996b, 1997). Throughout this chapter, the importance of evidence-based practice has been explored and related to the process of mentorship.

The importance of appreciating evidence-based practice

The emergence of clinical governance introduced by the government in 1997 and 1998 highlighted the importance of identifying best practice and the subsequent delivery of that best practice. According to FoNS (2001: 4), there were two main areas of focus encapsulated within clinical governance. This was to ensure that, 'evidence-based practice is supported and applied routinely in everyday practice' and 'programmes aimed at meeting the needs of individual health care professionals and the service needs of the organisation are in place and supported locally' (DH, 1998). A decade later, the use of evidence-based practice has now become the norm throughout healthcare and in the different stages throughout the patient's journey.

McEwan (2006a: 3) describes the influences that have changed and continue to change the approaches to nursing in contemporary healthcare. She states: 'Largely due to work of nursing scientists, nursing theorists and nursing scholars, over the past four decades, nursing has been recognised as both emerging profession and an academic discipline.' According to Banning (2005), the last decade has witnessed a transformation in nursing practice from being predominantly medically driven to one that is increasingly nurse-led. In order to ensure this development and change in nursing care delivery, nurses have to constantly update their knowledge and skills.

In support, Andalo (2006) reflects on a statement by Lynne Maher, Head of Innovation Practice at the National Health Service Institute for Innovation and Improvement, and emphasizes that nurses have a strong potential to influence change in the NHS. Maher argues that because nurses are the largest workforce in the NHS, they have the potential to identify areas of change and subsequently implement those changes in order to improve service delivery received by patients, their relatives and carers. Indeed, part of the NHS Institute's remit is to assist the NHS to meet appropriate government reforms (Andalo, 2006). However, this is not only pertinent to nursing and midwifery but also has an impact on the allied professions. Domain seven according to the NMC (2008a), reflects this proactive vision towards healthcare.

Evidence-based practice

The concept of evidence-based practice has appeared in nursing literature in the past few years and indicates a cognitive change in the delivery of nursing care. Some of the literature reviewed includes McEwan and Wills (2006) and Mason and Whitehead (2004) who highlight that this is viewed as an approach to problem-solving in clinical practice. McEwan (2006b) identifies four stages (see Box 8.1).

Box 8.1   Four main stages of problem solving

- Identifying a clinical problem.
- Searching the literature.
- Critically evaluating the research evidence.
- Determining appropriate interventions.

(McEwan, 2006b)

Mentors must therefore remember that the end result of evidence-based practice is the ability to offer research-based findings in order to justify aspects of care delivery and rationale for experiences encountered by patients throughout their healthcare journey in order to avoid bottlenecks and backlogs (NHS Institute for Innovation and Improvement, 2007). As a result, all healthcare students are encouraged to gain an awareness and appreciation of underpinning theoretical perspectives that validates the professional reputation associated with nursing, midwifery (NMC, 2008b) and the other allied professions (HPC, 2007a).

Brown (2008: 3) states, 'Effective nursing practice requires information, judgement, skills and art.' Hence, mentors must appreciate that the importance of evidence-based practice is to ensure that the care delivered to patients is research-based and not as a result of nursing rituals – 'that's the way that we have always done it on this ward'. Discussing domain seven with mentors at both mentor preparation and mentor updates indicates that there appears to be a generic belief in some healthcare settings that direct patient care is as a result of blasé statements, 'that's the way Sister likes it done', 'if it's not broken, why fix it?', 'it's worked for all these years – so why change now?' These statements may have had some credence in the past, but within the profession of contemporary nursing a more proactive stance is now becoming the norm. Burns and Grove (2007) highlight that this 'traditional' approach which is based on customs and trends can be restricting, narrow and can influence nursing practice.

Newell and Burnard (2006), Polit and Beck (2006), Burns and Grove (2007) and Brown (2008) all advocate the importance of nursing research as a fundamental approach to creating scientific knowledge that will emerge as a pioneer in establishing evidence-based nursing care. This is also supported by the NMC (2008b: 7) who state that nurses must 'provide a high standard of practice and care at all times' and in so doing, it is important to ensure that, 'you must deliver care based on the best available evidence or best practice'. Consequently, there is a need to review and appreciate the importance of clinical protocols, as these are regarded as standards of care that are pertinent to patients within the underlying guiding remit.

According to Brown (2008: 4), clinical protocols may be presented in the form of:

- Plans of care
- Standard order sets
- Clinical pathways
- Care algorithms
- Decision trees
- Bundles of recommended care actions and procedures.

Irrespective of the format, these approaches contribute to various aspects of evidence-based practice and should be used to guide healthcare professionals to deliver the care that has been deemed associated with the patient's needs. 'An appropriate committee or authority in the hospital, nursing department, or care-providing agency endorses each clinical protocol' (ibid.: 4). However, clinical protocols should only be used as a guide and therefore subsequently modified in order to meet the individualistic needs of the patient, resident or service user. They should be implemented according to need and altered if they are not achieving the desired outcome. Evidence-based nursing care is an approach that endeavours to deliver effective, personal and appropriate care to meet the recipient's individualistic needs. The mentor plays an important role in advocating research awareness (Box 8.2).

Box 8.2   Mentors advocating research awareness

The role of the mentor is to appreciate and gain an awareness of what research has been undertaken into the following three main components of mentorship:

1   Facilitation of learning.
2   Assessment and accountability.
3   Creating an environment for learning.

The role of the mentor is to support and assist healthcare students to understand the need for evidence-based practice as this will influence the three dominant themes of mentorship: facilitation of learning, assessment and creating an environment for learning. However, according to Castledine (2008), the process of nursing may be 'deteriorating'. He reports that there are two main problems within today's nursing profession. The first contrasts with the ideology underpinning evidence-based practice and that is, nurses don't seem to be bothered about aspects of patient care that involves meeting the fundamental personal needs and caring for people as individuals. The second problem he claims is that there is no continuity in the way that nurses approach their commitment to nursing practice. This he attributes to the changing culture of nursing that is evolving into a cosmopolitan profession in which there may be variation in acceptable standards. This criticism by Castledine (2008) emphasizes the potential dichotomy that exists between idealism and reality, creating a problem for the mentor when students ask them on what basis care is delivered in this placement.

However, Brown (2008: 10) highlights the pathway that a mentor may have to follow in order to appreciate the importance of evidence-based practice, this includes:

- Recognize when the nursing care being given is not as effective as it might be.
- Locate research-based guidelines and research summaries.
- Be comfortable reading research articles.
- Develop basic skills in judging if a clinical practice guideline or research summary was soundly produced.

- Decide if the research evidence available is strong enough to use as a basis for nursing care.
- Participate in the development of protocols in the agency or unit in which you work.

The aim of this chapter is to introduce the concept of evidence-based practice and to emphasize that in the pre-registration programme nursing students are also made aware of its significance. Therefore, when students arrive on placement they will expect their mentors to guide them in reading, understanding and applying research findings associated with the pertinent practice delivery.

There is now a plethora of literature that focuses on research in nursing, the research process, undertaking a research project and its implications for patient care. The mentor has to be aware of its importance in order to assist the student through their experience on that practice placement. It is not a mandatory component of mentorship to undertake a research project. However, it is important to be able to read a research-based article in order to increase the fundamental ideology of mentorship and how the process is evolving according to NMC (2008a), RCN (2007b), and HPC (2008) guidelines that attempt to mirror society's changing expectations of patient care and its relevance to healthcare students. It is important for mentors to be able to assess the quality of an article that their student may be reviewing in order to assist them to relate the identified theory to practice. Greenhalgh (1997, 2006) could be a useful approach (Box 8.3).

Box 8.3   A process for reviewing research-based literature

Greenhalgh (1997) considers five questions when reviewing a research-based article focusing on the following topics:

- the study;
- the research participants;
- the research design;
- the type of study;
- the importance of the research methodology.

Greenhalgh suggests that there are five questions that should be asked when reviewing a research-based article and as part of a literature review:

Question 1: Was the study original?

Ask the question: Does this new research add to the literature in any way?

Question 2: Whom is the study about?

Ask the questions:

- How were the subjects recruited?
- Who was included in the study?
- Who was excluded from the study?
- Were the subjects studied in 'real-life' circumstances?

Question 3: Was the design of the study sensible?

Ask the questions:

- What specific intervention or other manoeuvre was being considered, and what was it being compared with?
- What outcome was measured, and how?

Question 4: Was systematic bias avoided or minimized?

Ask the questions:

Was the design of the study a randomized controlled trial, a non-randomized comparative trial, a cohort study, or a case-control study?

Was assessment 'blind'? Even the most rigorous attempt to achieve a comparable control group will be wasted effort if the people who assess outcome know which group the research participant they are assessing was allocated to.

Question 5: Were preliminary statistical questions dealt with?

Ask the questions:

Three important numbers can often be found in the methods section of a paper: the size of the sample; the duration of follow-up; and the completeness of follow-up.

Was the study large enough, and continued for long enough, to make the results credible?

Students may be asked to undertake a literature review as an assignment in their nurse training, so knowing how to review an article in an identified format would be useful. On some post-registration degree programmes an optional written assignment could be an extended literature review. So the importance of evaluating research articles is significant from a number of perspectives although a number of other frameworks may be used.

Therefore, in order to help you value the importance of evidence-based practice, the chapter will explore:

1 The research process.
2 The provision of research-based evidence.
3 The implications of research for healthcare practice (Box 8.4).

Box 8.4   Evidence-based practice

The Research Process + Research Evidence + Implications for Healthcare Practice.

It is important that as a mentor you reflect on your existing knowledge gained during your student training or as a registered practitioner and identify how it can be related to these three main components. In Mentor Activity 8.1, this encourages you to reflect on your current knowledge and the significance that you actually attribute to the importance of research.

During this activity consider your personal and professional development and the impact that this has on your daily roles and responsibilities. Most mentors summarize this into three categories:

1 Manager
2 Leader
3 Teacher.

However, your discussion will depend on your speciality of healthcare and if you work in a hospital, community or independent-sector practice placement.

MENTOR ACTIVITY 8.1

Explore the importance of research applicable to your own specific aspect of healthcare.

What is its significance?

An increasing number of research articles are published that focus on the relationship between the mentor and the student which highlight the effectiveness of mentorship or areas for potential improvement. When reading Case study 8.1 reflect on and compare this scenario with your own mentorship style. Hopefully you appreciate that, despite research findings, your own and colleagues, reflections of mentorship can remain a positive and worthwhile experience.

CASE STUDY 8.1

A student made a complimentary comment regarding the mentor she had worked with on her last placement. She was completing an assignment based on a literature review and as part of the requirements had to discuss the research methodology utilized.

The student was pleasantly surprised to find out that her mentor had recently completed a post-registration module on evidence-based practice as part of her own Learning Beyond Registration degree programme. As part of that module, she also had to discuss the various approaches to research methodology.

So, not only was this mentor a very supportive and proactive person regarding adult nursing, she was also a valuable resource to help the student with her academic studies. The student was able not only to share her knowledge with the mentor but they both learnt from each other regarding the research process.

This was a valuable worthwhile experience for the student because the mentor was prepared to share her own academic learning rather than just her nursing expertise.

As a mentor how can you utilize your post-registration knowledge to enhance the student's learning?

The research process

Gerrish and McMahon (2006: 7) emphasize: 'Nurses who are research-aware will demonstrate the ability to find out about the latest research in their area together with an openness to change their practice when new knowledge becomes available.'

Mentors have to appreciate the significance of this statement and its implication for both patient care and mentorship awareness. Although some research is hard to undertake, Newell and Burnard (2006) identify that there are two fundamental reasons why it is important in contemporary healthcare:

- Research addresses an important question.
- It also identifies and responds to a gap in the literature.

This claim is supported by Polit and Beck (2006: 4) who state that, 'Research is systematic inquiry that uses disciplined methods to answer questions or solve problems. The ultimate goal of research is to develop, refine and expand a base of knowledge.' According to an ever increasing number of research–based literature sources, healthcare professionals are involved in researching into patient management and care delivery, and nurse education, including mentorship and nursing administration. Reflect back on Mentor Activity 8.1 and identify the importance that you give to research whilst undertaking your daily roles and responsibilities.

The Health Professions Council also emphasizes the importance of research. They state different ways in which allied professions can respond to research findings: Operating Department Practitioners: 'Registrants must be able to use research, reasoning and problem-solving skills (and, in the case of clinical scientists, conduct fundamental research)' (HPC, 2004: 11).

The Health Professions Council identifies the skills required for the application of practice. In Section 2b.1 they state that in the formulation and delivery of plans and strategies for meeting health and social care needs that Registrants must:

> Be able to use research, reasoning and problem-solving skills to determine appropriate actions:
>
> * recognize the value of research to the critical evaluation of practice;
> * be able to engage in evidence-based practice, evaluate practice systematically and participate in audit procedures;
> * be aware of a range of research methodologies;
> * be able to demonstrate a logical and systematic approach to problem solving;
> * be able to evaluate research and other evidence to inform their own practice. (HPC, 2007d; HPC, 2007f)

There are additional requirements, according to some professions:

> * be able to use statistical, epidemiological and research skills to gather and interpret evidence in order to make reasoned conclusions and judgements with respect to dietetic practice in disease prevention and management (HPC, 2007c);
> * recognize the need to discuss, and be able to explain the rationale for, the use of physiotherapy interventions;
> * be able to form a diagnosis on the basis of physiotherapy assessment (HPC, 2007e).

The importance of evidence-based practice is therefore pertinent to nursing, midwifery and the other allied professions as supported by both the NMC (2008a) and the HPC. However, the type of research can have an influence on its acceptance and applicability into the delivery of healthcare.

Types of research

There are three types of research that are identified in the numerous literature sources:

- qualitative;
- quantitative;
- combination of both qualitative and quantitative (Cormack, 2000; Polit and Beck, 2006; Newell and Burnard, 2006; Brown, 2008).

If a mentor is going to support evidence-based practice as advocated by the NMC (2008a) in domain seven, they will have to ensure they understand the difference between the two types. Some of the research articles that focus on mentorship favour one type but often utilize the combination type.

Examples

- 'Pre-registration student nurses' perception of the hospital-learning environment during clinical placements'. Midgley (2006) = quantitative research.
- 'Assessor or mentor? Role confusion in professional education', Bray and Nettleton (2007) = combination of qualitative and quantitative research.
- 'Changes in nurse education: Delivering the curriculum', Carr (2008) = qualitative research.
- 'Current mentorship schemes might be doing our students a disservice', Nettleton and Bray (2008) = combination of qualitative and quantitative research.
- '"I felt like a real nurse" – Student nurses out on their own', Anderson and Kiger (2008) = qualitative research.

Qualitative research

This type of research focus on a subjective approach involving what the participant says or writes down in a response to the way they think, feel and behave. Porter and Carter (2000: state, 19). 'Qualitative research is used as an umbrella term for those strategies that seek to explain human behaviour in terms of the reasons people have for behaving in the way they do.' This approach was used by all four researchers in the examples quoted and is the type chosen depending on the research question and what the researchers are investigating. Topping (2006) describes this as an interpretivist tradition in that in order to understand human behaviour, it needs to interpret interaction with others.

This research approach, 'strives to emphasise that there is no single interpretation, truth or meaning but recognise that just as human beings are different, so are the societies and cultures in which they live their lives' (ibid.: 158). The various data collection methods used to acquire qualitative data include in-depth conversations, diary keeping, extensive interviewing, extended observation, and focus groups to acquire insights regarding these subjective realities (Clarke and Iphofen, 2006; Brown, 2008).

The interview is perhaps the most popular research approach used to execute in-depth conversations. The approach can vary from the structured to the unstructured interview or as an alternative semi-structured. The structured interview can follow a set format but may not allow for any flexibility in the discourse. The unstructured interview often starts with a generalized open question from which the researcher can lead the proceeding conversation (Burnard, 2005; McCann and Clark, 2005; Walker, 2007).

Quantitative research

This approach differs as it is underpinned by a positivist tradition that proposes that scientific truths or laws exist (Topping, 2006). This is often called the scientific or empirical method because the methods used are objective and free from bias. Therefore, the data should be and are, 'untainted by the feelings, opinions or bias of the researcher or researched' (Porter and Carter, 2000: 142). The research data are collected by using questionnaires and therefore the information generated is numerical. Quantitative methods are used to test how well a nursing intervention works compared to another intervention.

On an individual basis, both qualitative and quantitative methods have their inherent advantages depending on the type of research question and the rationale for undertaking the research process. As a mentor, it is important that you appreciate the difference between the two approaches. However, this insight does no more than mention the difference between the two. As identified in the examples, researchers often adopt a combination approach by using both questionnaire (quantitative) and an interview approach (qualitative) (see Box 8.5). In order for you as a mentor to appreciate the importance of evidence-based practice, you need to adopt an unbiased approach so that you can review the two research methods. The importance of both methods is that they generate new knowledge that either contradicts existing understandings or provides data that previously didn't exist.

Box 8.5   Characteristics of quantitative and qualitative research

Quantitative research

- hard science
- objective
- political
- reductionist
- logico-deductive
- cause and effect relationships
- tests theory

- control
- instruments as data collection tools
- basic unit of analysis: numbers
- statistical analysis
- generalization

Qualitative research

- soft science
- subjective
- value-free
- holistic
- dialectic, inductive, speculative
- meaning
- develops, advances and re-interprets theory
- shared interpretation
- listening and talking, observation as ways of gathering data
- basic unit of analysis: words
- interpretation
- uniqueness/transferability

Source: Adapted from Burns and Grove (1997); Corner (1993); Silverman (2000), all cited in Topping (2006).

Box 8.5 summarizes the differences between both qualitative and quantitative research methods and subsequently what it is that makes them both important approaches in their own right. Irrespective of the approach taken, there is a need to consider the significance of ethics whilst undertaking a research study. Newell and Burnard (2006: 37) state: 'Health care ethics has undergone much change in the past few years, partly because of well-publicised cases of the abuse of patients and tissues from deceased patients in pursuit of research goals.' Consequently, the emphasis on protecting the research participant is stronger now than possibly it was in the past. Applying for and gaining ethical consent are now an important integral part of the research process.

Reflect on your understanding of the different research methods and complete Mentor Activity 8.2.

MENTOR ACTIVITY 8.2

Reflect on your own understanding of the differences between the two research approaches and identify which you think is the most appropriate for your area of healthcare.

Justify your choice.

In the various literature sources the actual research process does tend to vary although the fundamental approach is similar. In order to evaluate the effectiveness of any research findings, it is often necessary to undertake a literature review. This process entails examining each stage that the researcher has followed and has described in their research article, in order to achieve the resultant research data. The article will then allow the reader the opportunity to read through the stages and ascertain the effectiveness of the results attained. Complete Mentor Activity 8.3 to reflect on your own knowledge regarding the research process.

MENTOR ACTIVITY 8.3

What are the different stages in 'the research process'?

Make a list and then compare your answer with that proposed by Gerrish and Lacey.

The provision of research-based evidence

There are a number of stages in the research process that are systematically followed in order to achieve the end results: the research findings. Gerrish and Lacey (2006) describe these stages:

1 Development of the research question.
2 Searching and undertaking a literature review.
3 Identifying the research methodology/research design.
4 Preparing a research proposal.
5 Gaining access to the data.
6 Sampling.
7 Pilot study.
8 Data collection.
9 Data analysis.
10 Dissemination of results.
11 Implementation of results.

Researchers often follow the same stages in this framework, whilst others vary their approach in order to obtain the research data they are anticipating depending on whether they are using a qualitative or quantitative approach.

One qualitative approach relates to phenomenology, an attempt that encourages the participants to share their world with the researcher. Clarke and Iphofen (2006) state that phenomenology has become a very popular approach to nursing and other healthcare disciplines research, particularly in the past ten years. This research method attempts to understand human experience and hence its popularity for an understanding of the nature of nursing. It is regarded as both a philosophy and a methodology focusing upon the 'lived' experience of the individual and their intentions within the social world. Corben (1999) identifies that philosophy offers a vehicle for thinking about and answering questions pertinent to reality, truth and meaning but paradoxically warns of the complexities of the phenomeno-logical perspectives.

In understanding the mentor's experience of mentoring students or the student's experience of being mentored, phenomenology would be a valued approach because of its usefulness in helping understand human experiences. Phenomenology was first advocated by Edmund Husserl (1859–1935). Koch (1995) starts her explanation of the theory by relating to Cartesian duality, a model of the mind and the mind–body split, a mechanistic view of the person which was an influential theme in philosophy from Descartes (1598–1650) until Husserl. According to Koch (1995), it was on this basis that Husserl developed his idea of phenomenology so that it would be more meaningful. He proposed the concept of the 'life world' or 'lived experience', which argues that there is a need to re-examine taken-for-granted experiences. It could be argued that the mentor is taken for granted by their manager, educationalists and the students. Equally, men-toring as an activity could be overlooked by mentors who begin to treat it as 'second nature'.

However, it was the work of Martin Heidegger (1889–1976), a student of Husserl, who was acclaimed as the founder of modern hermeneutics, a second branch of phenomenology, which is different in important regards. His approach is founded on the ontological 'foundation of the understanding', which is obtained by 'being-in-the-world'. He clearly advocates the signif-icance of human everyday existence, by utilizing the term 'Dasein'. This is a conceptual term that emphasizes the importance of understanding 'what it is to be human', either from an individualistic or general perspective derived from our everydayness (Lindsay, 2006). Heideggerian approach is regarded as being less restrictive and could be applied to practice more effectively than the Husserlian approach (Table 8.1).

Therefore, using a Heideggerian approach does provide qualitative data that can then be appropriately analysed (Kinnell, 2004). There are other methods that could be utilized to obtain data and are equally advo-cated by other researchers. The use of open-ended questionnaires can generate qualitative data, providing that the questions are appropriately thought-provoking.

TABLE 8.1   *Heideggarian phenomenology: practical research implications*

Principle	Research implications
Knowledge	Co-created with the respondents. Knowledge is constructed through dialogue using the life experiences of both researcher and respondent.
Respondents	Co-researchers who discover personal meaning, their conception of the phenomenon with the researcher.
Researcher	A professional who sensitively cites the life world of the respondent using his or her own experiences as one of the tools.
Truth	Authentic accounts of a phenomenon as co-created by respondent and researcher.
Inquiry	Emic – getting inside the human experience.
Approach	Exploring phenomenon from within.

Use of questionnaires

Murphy–Black (2000: 301) states: 'A questionnaire can be used in different ways from the formal structured, completed by the respondents on their own, to the semi-structured interview completed with the researcher face-to-face.' The questionnaire is a vehicle for producing statistical data that can then be analysed and its significance related to the research question. One popular approach used is the postal questionnaire (Murphy–Black, 2000). This can be designed so that the participants are all asked the same question, in the same order, so that they can select and tick either 'yes', 'no', 'don't know', etc. in response to a constructive objective list of closed questions. Some questionnaires are designed using an open-ended question approach, which will then generate qualitative data. The design will depend on what type of information the researcher requires. Polit and Hungler (1999), Mathews and Chu Huang (2004) and Cohen and Manion (2007) highlight the importance of gaining data from questionnaires emphasizing the design of the research tool has to be effective in order to gain the desired response.

There are a number of advantages to completing a questionnaire such as the research participant can complete in their own home, at their own leisure, and at a time that is convenient to them, providing they are within the return date deadline. The returned completed questionnaires will provide data that can be correlated and analysed using a specific tool or programme. The numerical data gained from a closed question questionnaire can then be explored and its significance debated. An open-ended question design will need a different approach to its analysis.

Unfortunately, there are a number of disadvantages with using only a questionnaire, depending on the nature of the evidence that is anticipated. The success of using the questionnaire is dependent on the participant and how effective they answer the set questions (Cohen and Manion, 2007). Some problems include:

- The person may not answer the questions honestly or at all.
- The person may not be able to read and hence rely on someone else to help them complete the questionnaire.
- The person may misunderstand the question and inadvertently not provide the appropriate information.
- Some people do not like completing forms and may not take the time to provide the information required and hence there may be significant gaps.

The design of the questionnaire is important in order to attain the desired participant's response, according to Stommel and Wills (2004). Often a Likert scale is used as this guides the participants through the choices identified by the researcher. The Likert scale is an ordinal scale (Jordan et al., 1998), therefore a series of numbers appears in a systematic order (Fowler et al., 2002). The response rate and the quality of the resultant data will therefore depend on effectiveness of its design. Using questionnaires to gather data is usually economical, self-administered and can be distributed via mail or the internet.

Implications for healthcare practice

Regarding mentorship and the identified research-based articles the following is a synopsis of the research methods and tools used:

1   *Midgley (2006)* used a questionnaire which was formulated based on a list of preset statements that were either closed-questions or fixed alternatives using a Likert scale. The clinical-learning environment inventory (CLEI) developed by Chan (2001) was the research tool used in this study. The CLEI contains 42 statements with seven statements assessing each of six scales: personalization, student involvement, task orientation, innovation, satisfaction and individualization (which includes a relationship dimension; a personal dimension and a system maintenance and system change dimension). A cohort of second-year student nurses in acute hospital placements were selected as the sample population; 70 questionnaires were distributed and 67 were returned.

Implications for healthcare practice

The aim of this research was to identify a comparison between pre-registration student nurses' actual and preferred perceptions of the hospital learning environment with the clinical-learning environment inventory (CLEI) questionnaire that was used. The results of the scale showed that this particular cohort perceived satisfaction and personalization to be the most important domains in the hospital learning environment, closely followed by student involvement. The personalization scale addressed the opportunities for each learner to interact with their mentor and members of the nursing team and on concern for students' personal welfare.

Midgley found that the greatest difference between how student nurses found the learning environment to be and how they would prefer it to be was in the area of innovation. The statistics imply that in comparison with the actual hospital environment, students would prefer an environment with higher levels of individualization, innovation in teaching and learning strategies, student involvement, personalization and task orientation. A fundamental principle and expectation of nurse education and training are the preparation of the learner for a professional role. The clinical field provides a unique and pivotal role in this preparation, according to Midgley.

2   *Bray and Nettleton (2007)* used a questionnaire which was distributed by post to midwifery, medical and nursing mentors based in five acute trusts. The questionnaires were also distributed to midwifery, medical and nurse mentees during lectures/ seminars and via the post. The questionnaires sought to obtain both quantitative and qualitative data focusing on the level of mentor training, difficulties experienced in the role, perceptions of a 'good' mentor and experiences of acting as a mentor.

Implications for healthcare practice
The aims of the study were to explore:

- How is mentoring conceptualized in the health setting?
- Which factors influence the mentor–mentee relationship in a positive/ negative way?
- What are the professional and personal needs of the mentees?
- What are the training and development needs of mentors?

   (Bray and Nettleton, 2007: 850)

The research found that there was still some confusion related to the process of mentorship, the inter-changeable definitions and role titles that are used in the contemporary healthcare culture. The study involved nursing, midwifery and medicine and the results identified that mentors viewed assessment as less of a priority, compared to the more supportive pastoral role and the importance of sharing clinical knowledge and skills. It was emphasized by Bray and Nettleton that assessment or appraisal should not be a part of the mentorship process as this complicates the supportive partnership. Hence, there appears some role confusion between what constitutes a mentor and an assessor.

3   *Carr (2008)* based his research on 37 in-depth interviews with nurse teachers. The transcripts were subject to a content analysis framework for qualitative data analysis.

The participants made 59 qualitative comments identifying significant changes in nursing education. Three themes emerged: the nature of nursing has changed (25%), the selection of future nurses is problematic (34%) and the current large numbers of students are straining the fabric of the nursing education system (41%).

Implications for healthcare practice

Some of the main issues identified how 'nursing' continues to evolve and be transformed in its quest to substantiate the claim that it is a research-based profession. Carr examined the transcripts from the interviews and presents brief quotes in order to emphasize the qualitative data obtained. He emphasized that the culture of nursing is changing and asks if the label 'nurse' must not be as appropriate for healthcare workers undertaking nursing work. This was accentuated by the acknowledgement that contemporary nurses engage more in undertaking managerial functions that are often combined with advanced technical skills.

However, this change in roles and responsibilities perhaps offers the nurse more scope to develop their knowledge, skills and attitudes. This article clearly advocates a change in the nurse's role. The student selection is problematic because the entry gate into nursing has been widened and this has inherent challenges. Carr (2008: 123) states: 'Students who lack confidence in their literary and numeric skills find the transition to the higher education difficult and they rightly seek support from the nurse teachers employed to help them.' The increase in number of student nurses per intake was also seen as problematic for both education and placement providers.

4 *Anderson and Kiger (2008)* used a qualitative approach to discover the experiences of student nurses working on their own in the community and what these experiences meant to them. The research question was: 'What are the experiences of student nurses who undertake unsupervized visits to deliver care to patients and clients in the home setting?' A semi-structured format was used with the interviews being tape-recorded.

Implications for healthcare practice

In response to the one-to-one interviews, the following component themes justified why the students felt 'like a real nurse' including 'building confidence', 'developing professionalism in relationships', 'learning to manage care', 'developing knowledge and gaining insight' and 'being included and supported'. The value of this study was that it contributed to the meaning that these students attached to the experience of independent working and how they were developing as sense of professionalism in readiness for completing their own nurse training programme.

These summaries are included to emphasize to mentors the importance of research in order to generate new knowledge that doesn't yet exist. Alternatively, research studies serve to criticize and update existing knowledge, hence the importance of evidence-based practice in contemporary healthcare. Research into mentorship is valued because it helps to understand the role of both the mentor and the mentee within the supportive partnership. Both the NMC and the HPC support the significant role of research to develop the existing epistemology related to healthcare and the creation of new knowledge. The mentor has to appreciate the diversity of their professional role and the significance of research in improving the components of that role as manager, leader and teacher.

The mentor is presented with a number of challenges by their healthcare student, whether it is an intra-personal or inter-personal issue. Throughout their experience on your placement they may be asked to produce a Student Portfolio of evidence (NMC, 2004c: 34) although this may not be pertinent to all allied professions. The Student Portfolio is certainly problematic for some students but yet it is important. The NMC (2004c: 34) states that students should 'demonstrate responsibility for one's own learning through the development of a portfolio of practice and recognise when further learning is required'. Whatever the student needs to achieve in their practice placement, the mentor can be a reassuring and positive influence on the student's progress. Read Case study 8.2 for a successful approach to mentorship.

CASE STUDY 8.2

A student nurse described the support and guidance that she was given whilst on her first placement, when trying to produce a selection of evidence to meet her practice placement outcomes. She said that her mentor had identified her specific strengths and weaknesses at her initial interview before constructing a realistic action plan. The student said she found the overall experience of her first placement overwhelming because of her limited nursing experience. However, her mentor had been empathic, encouraged her to 'think for herself' but yet gave her positive feedback when appropriate.

She found the thought of the Essential Skills Cluster Assessments daunting because they were a summative assessment but yet the mentor had talked her through the assessment criteria and what she expected of her. Subsequently, she successfully passed two of the assessments which she was pleased with.

In her discussion, the student reiterated that although she was learning basic nursing skills, the mentor was a strong influence on her learning, which she felt had given her the confidence for her next practice placements. Consider a positive mentorship experience you have been involved in – why was it so successful?

These are just a few examples of research into mentorship and emphasize that over the past 20 years, the interest continues to escalate (Myall et al., 2008). Since its origin associated with Project 2000 (UKCC, 1986) whereby student nurses were given supernumerary status, mentorship has become a respected role that most qualified staff aspire to attain. The role of mentorship is now incorporated into job descriptions and is an important requirement or necessity if qualified staff wish to move up the promotional ladder. Myall et al. (2008: 1841) stated that the findings of their research confirmed 'that mentorship in contemporary nursing practice remains integral to students' clinical experiences and that it has a significant influence on the quality of their placements, the sense of "connectedness" they experience and their learning'. It is anticipated that whilst working with their mentor, the student will develop the knowledge, skills and attitudes that are required for them to be effective on registration.

Moore (2005), an independent consultant, produced a policy review that examined to what extent nurse education prepared students in order to ensure their fitness for practice at the point of registration. This was in response to concerns regarding the effectiveness and competence of newly qualified nurses. A Nursing Task and Finish Group was commissioned by the Nursing and Midwifery Council to examine approaches taken by other health regulators in the United Kingdom, and nurse regulators in other English-speaking countries, to explore how effective newly qualified nurses are once they gain their registration. The final report did not find any 'evidence of systematic failure to prepare nurses who are fit for practice at the point of registration' (Moore, 2005: 21). However, the main area of concern related to the process of assessment, a concern that had already been highlighted by Duffy (2004).

The Policy Review also stated that:

> The mentor role is absolutely pivotal to practice-based learning and assessment. There are inconsistencies and weaknesses in the preparation and support of mentors and difficulties in ensuring that there are sufficient mentors to accommodate the recent growth in student numbers. (Moore, 2005: 23)

The NMC (2008a) clearly identifies that mentor training should be a ten-day programme, five days protected time and five days related to work-based learning. Hence, the importance of this policy review has influenced the way of contemporary mentor training.

Throughout this chapter the significance of evidence-based practice has been explored not from a direct patient care, delivery or management perspective but significantly has shown how mentorship is and has also developed its own catalogue of research-based findings. The interest in mentorship continues to initiate research studies involving either the effectiveness of the mentor or the behaviour of the student. The different approaches and research methodologies can be applied depending on the final result required. Some researchers use a quantitative approach in order to produce significant statistical, objective evidence. Others utilize more of a qualitative approach in order to generate thoughts and feelings and hence a subjective overview. However, despite this increasing epistemology, the challenges still arise as indicated in the next section of Frequently asked questions.

Frequently asked questions

Mentors

Q. Why do some students think that they only have to achieve the competency, outcome or proficiency once? Surely, once achieved they should want to continue to develop the skill and apply it to different patients in order to become proficient?

A. When students are asked this question, they reiterate that they must achieve all the NMC (2004c) requirements and those in the branch programme, and that involves a lot of proficiencies. Once they have met the basic requirements, they state that they feel safe. However, it is up to the mentor to decide what is required in order to verify that the student has achieved what is expected of them, according to their level of training. If this entails more direct observations, it is within the mentor's remit to request that practice-based evidence. It is anticipated that the knowledge, skills and attitudes developed in one practice placement should be able to be transferred to another healthcare setting.

Q. I worked with a student who just didn't appear to be interested. She was late for duty and appeared to lack motivation, enthusiasm or willingness to learn. How am I supposed to effectively mentor a student like her?

A. The lateness for duty must be discussed, and if it does not improve must be documented in the student's Final Interview Report. The student's apparent lack of interest, motivation, and enthusiasm must be discussed with her and your concerns documented. The mentor needs to try and encourage the student to develop their evidence- or research-based awareness and link this knowledge to any assessments or written assignments that they may be currently involved with. If no improvement is made, you must inform your manager and educational link or follow the local guidelines in the Mentor Framework if available. You need to explore some of the more recent research-based literature sources that explore why students behave the way that they do.

Students

Q. Why do some mentors treat all students the same? They seem to have forgotten how 'nervous' we are when we first start a placement – a little more consideration would be appreciated. Is that a lot to ask?

A. This is an issue that students must discuss with their mentors as part of the orientation and initial interview. Sometimes the mentor needs to be told how students feel in order for them to be empathic. Mentors are encouraged to maintain their credibility and mentorship currency by ensuring that their own knowledge and awareness of the student's training programme reflect the current trend. As part of mentorship and particularly the orientation of students into practice, mentors are encouraged to examine any research-based articles in order that they can support their practice more effectively.

Q. My mentor keeps changing her shift at the last minute when we were supposed to be working together. She doesn't always tell me, so how am I supposed to ensure that the knowledge that I am gaining is evidence-based in order to meet my placement outcomes?

A. Unfortunately, mentors sometimes have to change their duty rota at the last minute to encompass sickness, staffing problems, personal problems or cover night duty. Your mentor should try and keep you informed and arrange for someone to mentor you if they do change their duty rota. If a student is concerned about the quality of their evidence-based knowledge, they must identify the topic specifically related to individual staff members. These staff members usually have a personal interest in a specific topic and may have developed and maintain an up-to-date folder of significant evidence-based articles of interest that the student can read or use to help them develop their research awareness.

Chapter summary

The overall content of this chapter has focused on the importance of evidence-based practice and its impact on the process of mentorship. Having completed this chapter you have learned about:

- the emergence of evidence-based practice and its now established role within healthcare delivery;
- the mentor's role in evaluating evidence-based research findings and how to support healthcare students in appreciating its significance in contemporary healthcare;
- the difference between qualitative and quantitative research findings and how they may influence mentorship;
- the importance of data collections and the different research methods that are utilized;
- the application of evidence-based practice in understanding the different expectations of mentorship from the mentor and mentee perspectives.

Further reading

Brown, S.J. (2008) *Evidence-Based Nursing: The Research-Practice Connection*. London: Jones and Bartlett Publishers.

This is a really useful text that explores the ever increasing awareness of the diversity of the research process, methods and methodology. The relevance of research in emphasizing the importance of evidence-based practice is a significant theme identified throughout.

Gerrish, K. and Lacey, A. (eds) (2006) *The Research Process in Nursing*, 5th edn. Oxford: Blackwell Publishing.

This is a compilation of 33 chapters produced by different authors. The book follows the research process and is divided into six significant parts, each exploring an aspect of the process effectively.

9

Leadership:

An integrated role within mentorship

David Kinnell
Philip Hughes

Nursing and Midwifery Council (2008a): Eight domains of mentorship
Domain Eight: Leadership

Aim

Demonstrate leadership skills for education within practice and academic settings.

Outcomes

Stage 1: Nurses and Midwives

- Use communication skills effectively to ensure that those in learning experiences understand their contribution and limitations to care delivery.

Stage 2: Mentor

- Plan a series of learning experiences that will meet students' defined learning needs.
- Be an advocate for students to support them accessing learning opportunities that meet their individual needs, involving a range of other professionals, patients, clients and carers.

(Continued)

(Continued)

- Prioritize work to accommodate support of students within their practice roles.
- Provide feedback about the effectiveness of learning and assessment in practice.

The importance of domain eight is implicit in the overeaching aim and the associated supporting outcomes for both Stage One and Stage Two mentors. The domain encompasses a need to review communication strategies but also the effectiveness of managing learning and assessment in the practice placement and academic setting. The process of leadership has been explored from a number of perspectives, both past and present, the basic principles have been incorporated into domain eight and are inherent in pre-registration students' management semesters or final placements before registration. Student nurses are prepared for their role as a leader, manager and a teacher and these three prerequisites are often emphasized in the job descriptions that they strive to correlate to, in order to successfully attain their first post as a qualified nurse.

Introduction

Leadership is an integrated role that mentors have to undertake whilst also executing their mentorship skills. The importance of being an effective leader correlates to the importance of being acknowledged and respected for the commitment that mentors show to ensuring that healthcare students gain the most from their practice placements. There is some benefit in reflecting on existing underpinning theoretical perspectives regarding leadership and its alliance with mentorship though there is some disparity in the way that mentors actually meet all the requirements that are expected of them. The NMC (2008a) has implemented changes that will have an impact now and in the future as mentors respond to those recommendations.

Leadership within healthcare

Leadership skills are an integrated feature throughout any healthcare student's training surreptitiously, as they manage their time, balancing practice experience with their academic requirements and assessments. Throughout the duration of their training, students will inevitably experience times when, on reflection, they realize that their time management was not as effective as it could have been. At the end of a busy shift, the mentor may well reflect on their experience of the day and realize that the time could have been managed more productively. However, the mentor's role is forever changing, as they are expected to be a coordinator of patient care, a care manager, an expert in their own clinical field and if that isn't enough, they are also expected to teach and assess healthcare students within their commitment to mentorship.

The literature emphasizes this ever changing perception of leadership and what this role entails as reflected in various definitions of what the process entails. According to Kenmore (2008: 25), there are a number of leadership styles including:

- *directive* in which there is immediate compliance;
- *visionary* involved in providing long-term directions and vision;
- *affiliative* which relates to creating harmony;
- *participative* involving developing staff commitment and generating ideas;
- *pace-setting*, accomplishing tasks to high standards;
- *coaching* which involves the long-term professional development of staff.

Healthcare professionals, nurses, midwives and other allied professions will have their own expectations of what leadership is and which qualities and skills make a good leader. This is particularly pertinent for the Stage One mentor as they start the career that they have just spent three years training for.

With the transition into their leadership role, they will become a member of the mentorship team. Each member works in a team in order to ensure the student's experience of mentorship is as positive as can be achieved. The mentorship team could include:

- the registered Stage Two mentor;
- the associate/co-mentor (who may be a Stage One mentor) who contributes by working and supporting the student in the absence of the main mentor and assists in the construction of the Student Portfolio of evidence.

Consider this plan of the student's learning experiences (see Box 9.1).

Box 9.1   A plan of the student's practice learning experiences

Week 1

- Welcome and introduce student to the placement, the mentorship team, other staff members and patients.
- Complete:

(Continued)

(Continued)

    (a)   Orientation – show the student around the geography of the practice placement including staff room and facilities, changing area, fire exits, emergency call buzzer, answering the telephone, etc.

    (b)   Initial interview – complete the first interview, identify the student's expectations and aspirations, correct any misconceptions they may have regarding the placement. Discuss if there were any weaknesses identified on the last placement and the action plan that was written in the Ongoing Achieving Record.

- Identify placement learning outcomes or proficiencies and how they will be achieved at the student's level of training.
- Identify if the student has any essential skills clusters assessments to complete or OSCEs to prepare for. Discuss how you will plan to assist them achieve these requirements.
- Ask the student if they have any related written academic assignments that they have to complete and may need advice on, whilst on the practice placement.

Weeks 2–3

- Assist student to achieve outcomes or proficiencies by offering advice on the range of evidence to collect and how to complete Student Portfolio.
- Maintain a continuous assessment approach ascertaining student's progress, strengths and weaknesses.
- Clarify the range of healthcare experiences that are related to the placement.
- Assist the student to start making the link between theory and practice.
- Discuss with the mentorship team the student's progress.

Weeks 3–4

- Complete the intermediate interview highlighting progress made and the academic requirements that need to be achieved.
- Must compliment on progress before specifying areas of concerns.
- Discuss how the mentor wants to manage this situation and if the academic link needs to be involved.
- Construct an action plan on how the deficits can be achieved and involve the mentorship team.
- Ascertain if the student is ready to complete their essential skills cluster assessment – establishing which one, arranging the date and time.
- Ensure the student is starting to understand the placement speciality of patient care, theory and practice.
- What insight visits are pertinent to the placement, have they attended and completed an observed learning/insight visit statement (or equivalent) highlighting what they have learnt and the outcomes/proficiencies achieved.

Weeks 4–5

- Monitor the student's progress, offer advice and guidance as required.
- Any areas of concern must be discussed with the student and you seek advice from the academic link. A written record must be maintained of your concerns according to your local policy.
- Continue to verify the outcomes or proficiencies as they are achieved on a weekly basis.
- If the student lacks motivation, interest and enthusiasm, this must be discussed with the individual so that they can improve their intrapersonal and interpersonal communication skills.
- Discuss with the mentorship team the development of the student.
- Undertake any essential skills clusters placement assessments.

Weeks 5–6

- Discuss with the team the student's progress.
- Complete the student's Ongoing Achievement Record, verifying the outcomes or proficiencies achieved.
- Identify the outcomes or proficiencies not achieved and state why this was a problem: no opportunity, insufficient evidence, unsafe practice, etc.
- Undertake the final interview and provide the student with constructive feedback.
- Specify any areas of weakness and construct an action plan for the next placement – record this in the student's Ongoing Achievement Record.
- Ensure that all the documentation is complete and the student takes this with them when they leave the practice placement.
- The mentor and associate mentor need to record that they have mentored this student as part of their triennial review record.

It is envisaged that this structure will enhance a series of learning experiences that will assist student nurses to meet their defined learning needs. The effectiveness of that experience may be enhanced by other members of the placement staff as well as other students who contribute to the mentorship team. In their final management semester, third-year students are encouraged to gain an insight into being a mentor by acting as a 'buddy'. This is the role of a third-year student supporting more junior students, sharing their expertise and allaying fears. The term will vary according to the higher educational institute but the 'buddy system' is one version.

The 'buddy' system or equivalent – valuing the role of senior students

This is a supportive mechanism that has been used in some higher educational institutes since its introduction into nurse training in 2000. It could be argued that nursing operates a similar system under a different name but the underpinning idea is the same. The concept behind this or similar systems is that a third-year student nurse would gain an insight into the facilitation of learning and create an environment for learning, capitalizing and further developing the experiences that they had experienced throughout their journey since commencing nurse training. This is also regarded as a prerequisite to becoming an associate mentor. The buddy system (also known as the peer support system) could be further developed in order to meet the more recent changes in both practice and in nurse education. If this is not already in existence, perhaps this could be incorporated in order to enhance mentorship.

The third-year student could then be introduced to the role of Stage One mentor and prepared to meet the outcomes following their registration. Indeed, a programme could be established whereby the student would attend a three-day Stage One mentor preparation course in which they could explore and discuss the eight domains of mentorship and the overall 14 outcomes associated with the Stage One level in the developmental framework. If this was adopted, it could create an opportunity for students to examine their future roles and responsibilities before they gain their registration – consider the feasibility of such a short training programme.

The buddy could also focus on helping the junior student prepare for their essential skills clusters summative assessment and therefore be a supportive staff member. The role is predominantly related to nursing, and helping prepare junior students for their practice assessments, although the buddy is not directly involved in the assessment function of mentorship. Those students who have experienced this support mechanism reflect on this as a positive experience.

The general aims of the buddy system are:

- to reduce students anxiety in new placements;
- to help students to acquire essential care skills;
- to help students to integrate theory with practice, encourage the skills of reflection alongside more experienced students. (Aston, 2005)

Guidelines for mentors wishing to implement the buddy system are:

Senior students:

- ensure the senior student's clinical skills are of a high standard;
- support the senior student who is buddying – give them advice on what is appropriate to undertake;
- give constructive feedback to the senior student.

Junior students:

- ascertain that the junior student is developing essential care skills and practising them safely prior to the essential skills clusters assessments;
- ensure that the junior student gets feedback from the mentor as well as the buddy regarding their overall development;
- monitor whether the person being 'buddied' is becoming more relaxed and confident in their nursing skills (Aston, 2005).

A friendly healthcare assistant – a valued contribution to mentorship

A friendly healthcare assistant (or equivalent title) could contribute to the mentorship process by sharing their fundamental knowledge of the placement management and daily routine with nursing students who are new to the placement. The knowledge and skills of the healthcare assistant can now be valued as a contribution to helping the student get the most from their placements. Already in existence but not by the same name, they can be a vital linchpin in the orientation process by doing the following:

- undertaking a guided tour for the 'new' student and discussing how the ward or department operates;
- explaining day-to-day routine;
- helping at visiting times;
- helping at operating theatre days for patient surgery general and minor operations;
- contributing to helping the student develop practical skills – hygiene, toileting, feeding, mouth care, etc.;
- they do not have a role in assessment but may offer constructive comments to the Stage Two mentor.

In some practice placements the mentorship team may comprise four people who work together to facilitate learning, assess the effectiveness of that learning and creating and sustaining an effective environment for learning. The benefits of this 'mentorship team' (see Box 9.2) relates to the team dynamics and cohesion, as well as ensuring that the student will have someone to relate to in the absence of their registered mentor. However, this is an idealistic approach which is not always possible to achieve in small teams and is dependent on the availability of all four staff members. Some practice placements may have a similar process but identified by different titles. Reflect on your own practice environment and consider this as an area for improvement.

Box 9.2   The mentorship team

The team

- the Stage Two registered mentor
- the associate or co-mentor (who may be a Stage One mentor)
- the 'buddy'
- the 'friendly healthcare assistant'.

As identified, one of the main attributes required by a Stage Two mentor is effective leadership skills which are required both for managing their practice area as well as ensuring the student follows their identified series of learning experiences. The specific insight visits will be determined by the speciality of nursing and it is up to the student to arrange following discussion with their mentor. To allow you a chance to reflect on your own experiences, complete Mentor Activity 9.1.

MENTOR ACTIVITY 9.1

What do you consider are the qualities and skills needed to be an 'effective' leader?

Reflect on this question before continuing.

This is a question that has been examined and subsequently described by Pettinger (2007), so compare your answer with his. In addition to intra-personal variables, an effective leader will adopt their own preferred style of leadership and this may differ according to the individual's personality, the remit of their professional roles and responsibilities which are pertinent to the area of healthcare. There are a number of leadership styles that you may relate directly to or maybe your style is a combination, depending on the situation that you have to lead and manage.

Styles of leadership

There are a number of well-established and documented leadership styles including autocratic, consultative, democratic, and laissez-faire as some examples (Pettinger, 2007).

Autocratic (tyrannical) style

In this approach the philosophy is 'do as you are told' and hence the leader makes the decisions, supervises the subordinates without their consultation, or consideration for their opinion. The environment can be one of control where conformity is demanded. This may appear to be a well-organized placement to the onlooker but it is not necessarily one that is conducive for learning for healthcare students. Indeed, in their student evaluation of placement feedback, students have reported practice placements that appear to adhere to these principles and how they were made to feel de-valued and their opinions were squashed when they offered information regarding recent evidence-based practice research findings. This type of placement could make mentorship problematic when trying to enhance the Nursing and Midwifery Council's (2008a) recommendations.

This style of leadership, it could be argued, 'gets the job done'. The subordinates or team members know where they stand and directions or tasks are made clear. However, this style is not necessarily participative and so is dependent solely on the skills of the leader or manager. This style does have its good points as it is useful when dealing with an emergency situation, the leader directing the other members to undertake their assigned role within the established team approach.

Consultative/participative style

This is one of the more successful approaches to leadership that is pertinent to a wider number of healthcare settings. In this style the leader consults with the staff, and usually has a good rapport and communication with others. The leader is supportive and encourages questions. They tend to be more approachable, but at the same time retain their responsibility and are accountable for the results. The advantage of this style is that the final decision is objective and has a utilitarian end result. Mentorship is accepted into the practice placement and staff can share their views as to ascertaining the most effective way of meeting the Nursing and Midwifery Council's (2007a) requirements – the assessments of the essential skills clusters, for example.

This seems to be the more acceptable style in that it includes and values subordinate individuals without the leader evading their role and responsibility. However, there could be a price to pay for this style in that arguments or debates could take over and cause delay in reaching the required objectives. This style does encourage communication and can therefore reduce friction and frustration at these times of debate.

Democratic/participative style

This is a leadership style adopted in a number of healthcare settings whereby managerial decisions are decided by the team, on a democratic voting approach. There is an equal opportunity for all staff to contribute and the final decisions are usually as a result of consensus opinion. The leadership is assumed by a chairperson who reflects, summarizes and advertises the final decision made by the majority of the team. Mentorship is a team approach, so any issues, changes in assessment strategy or the educational curriculum can be discussed and any amendments decided by the team.

This approach does enhance intrapersonal and interpersonal communication skills as well as strengthening group cohesion. Students are welcomed into the practice placements and their contributions respected and discussed, consequently, they feel 'part' of that team. Therefore, within this democratic approach the leader's role is reduced and the team is subsequently 'team led'. The possibility of fragmentation and a lack of clear direction can be experienced, often leading to dissatisfaction among the subordinate or team members.

Laissez-faire style

This leadership style is appropriate for some practice placements but for others would be viewed as problematic. The overall approach is one that is very relaxed, lacks structure and has a tendency to let the subordinates 'get on with things'. Depending on the healthcare speciality, this lack of structure and unorganized approach could lead to a style of mentorship that the student may find disturbing because it does not correlate to the experiences they have found advantageous on other placements. However, the style is pertinent in some healthcare settings and develops appropriate teamwork when this leadership style has been well established.

This approach could be seen as a further move towards a team's self-management. This can happen where the leader lets people 'get on with things' but does not necessarily want to take responsibility for the outcomes. It is possible that this style can work where subordinates are clear in their role and well motivated as a team. It is important that the manager is still seen as the manager and leader, accepting responsibility for targets or outcomes. The manager could also adopt an advisory or consultative role.

Pettinger (2007) identifies a leadership continuum with 'boss-centred' leadership, where use of authority by the manager, on one hand, and on the other, 'subordinate-centred' leadership where there is an area of freedom used for subordinates. There is a range of behaviours:

Autocratic	Consultative
Production-centred	Employee-centred
Close	General
Initiating structure	Consideration
Task-directed	Human Relations
Directive	Supportive
Directive	Participative

FIGURE 9.1 *The leadership spectrum*
Source: (Pettinger, 2007).

- Manager makes decision and announces it.
- Manager 'sells' decision.
- Manager presents ideas and invites questions.
- Manager presents tentative decision subject to change.
- Manager presents problem, gets suggestions, makes decision.
- Manager defines limits, asks group to make decision.
- Manager permits subordinates to function within limits defined by supervisor.

Each leadership style has its positive and negative characteristics. Reviewing Pettinger's (2007) 'leadership continuum', it could be argued that there are a number of issues that are significant within the process of mentorship (Figure 9.1). A mentor should have insight into the different leadership styles and evaluate the one that appears to be dominant within their practice placement and how that style could influence the healthcare student's experience. A student could be viewed as a malleable commodity that needs to be exposed to a successful leadership style so that when qualified, they too could adopt that approach. Some mentors may argue that their particular approach to leadership does not necessarily belong to one particular label. They have adopted an amalgamation of the different styles according to the need, the situation and the individuals that they encounter. The art of good leadership or management is bringing out the best in people in order to accomplish the team directives, goals and specific outcomes.

The qualities and skills of an 'effective leader' as identified in Mentor Activity 9.1 may include the following:

- Someone who has underpinning theoretical perspectives associated with the psychology of leadership and applies that knowledge appropriately.
- Knowledgeable in own clinical area and associated nursing expertise.
- Patience and the need for repetition if required.
- Good insight and able to demonstrate effective interpersonal communication skills.
- The application and understanding of the effect of their particular leadership style and its influences on staff and students.
- Personal attributes – approachable, honest and straightforward.

- A clear understanding and application of the individuality of learning, theory and style.
- An up-to-date knowledge of the student's training programme.
- Knowing when to seek help or support from colleagues, or academic staff.

A number of these leadership attributes are applied throughout *The Code for Nurses and Midwives* (NMC, 2008b) and the guidelines for registrants, the standards of conduct, performance and ethics stated by the Health Professions Council (HPC, 2008). Irrespective of the specialism of the healthcare student, they can all encounter mentors who demonstrate effective leadership skills, but unfortunately the converse may also be experienced. In domain eight, the Stage Two mentor needs to ensure that students of nursing and midwifery gain an awareness of interprofessional learning, hence the need to value the similarity between both the NMC and the HPC.

The NHS Institute for Innovation and Improvement (2006) identify in their framework three main clusters – personal qualities, setting direction and delivering the service. The 'personal qualities' of a leader should focus on their self-belief, self-awareness, self-management, drive for improvement and personal integrity. These all relate to the qualities and skills that make an effective mentor, identified by potential mentors and student nurses. In the 'setting direction' cluster the NHS Institute identifies important areas as seizing the future, intellectual flexibility, broad scanning, political astuteness and drive for results. In contrast the third cluster 'delivering the service' explores the importance of leading change through people, holding the account, empowering others, effective and strategic influencing and collaborative working. The importance of the mentor's role is to balance these requirements with those of being a 'teacher' in the practice setting, facilitating and assessing the student's learning appropriately.

Jones (2008b) discusses 'Leadership in the "new" NHS' and the importance of appreciating that nurses may have the opportunity to develop their leadership skills. She states: 'Safe and effective clinical practice cannot be ensured unless nurses are effective managers and leaders at all levels of service delivery' (ibid.: 32). As a result of changes within the contemporary NHS with an emphasis focused on interprofessional learning, nurses will have to update their leadership and management skills to correspond to changing expectations.

Some of the characteristics of nursing's future role, stated by Jones (2008b), include:

- Contribution to health and healthcare at all levels.
- Ensuring a spirit of openness, mutual appreciation and collaboration between health and other care professionals and patients, or clients, and their families.

- Working in partnerships across sectors of health and social care, and taking responsible, visible roles.
- Working as members of integrated teams, to lead, to follow, in non-hierarchical multiprofessional and multi-agency systems.
- Working effectively in changing contexts, and managing change processes effectively.

In this review of nursing and its potential managerial future there is the re-emergence of the need to effectively manage change. Since the transition from the United Kingdom Central Council for Nursing, Midwifery and Health Visiting to the Nursing and Midwifery Council in 2002, the nursing profession has been subject to a number of changes in order to assist the profession in its quest to be recognized as a research-based profession. Mentors are not strangers to change as they have to respond to both practice-based and academic-specific changes.

Allan et al. (2008) in their literature study for learning in the clinical practice identify a number of significant literature sources that explore the concept of leadership for learning in British healthcare settings. Their foundation is influenced by the changes in ward management since the inception of the NHS Plan (DH, 2000). The associated changes have had an impact not only on ward management and its associated nursing practice but also on nurse education.

Consider your existing experiences as you complete Mentor Activity 9.2.

MENTOR ACTIVITY 9.2

What contribution can you make as a mentor to improving the practice placement?

How could you implement an aspect of change within your practice placement in order to improve the learning environment?

What factors would prevent you from implementing that aspect of change?

Consider these questions before continuing.

Clark (2008: 30) states, 'Effective clinical leadership is essential in delivering the high-quality, person-centred envisioned by health minister Lord Darzi in the final report of the NHS Next Stage Review, *High Quality Care for All* (Department of Health (DH) 2008).' The next section focuses on the impact of managing change.

Managing change

Mentors occupy a significant role in responding to both Department of Health and Nursing and Midwifery Council reforms and need to identify the most effective ways that change in the NHS can be implemented. In order to be effective, it is important to understand how change can be introduced, the stages of implementing change, the challenges that may be encountered and how group cohesion may be instrumental in establishing the success of any changes in service delivery. Whyte (2007) highlights the importance of teams working together to achieve their departmental aims and objectives identified within their philosophy of care. It must be remembered that some of the changes introduced within the contemporary NHS are intended to improve the patient's journey through their healthcare experience.

It could be argued that some of these NHS changes are deliberate and in response to a government recommendation from the Department of Health. This type of change is called *planned change* (Iles and Sutherland, 2001; Menix, 2003) and mentors are asked to contribute to its implementation. However, an alternative method of change is described as emergent change and this would evolve out of reviewing existing nursing practice, assessment of patient care effectiveness, audit review of the feedback received from patients who have used the service and subsequently identified potential areas for change.

Change is an important perspective if the NHS is to continually develop to meet contemporary healthcare needs. Academic changes are introduced as a result of changing expectations that patients and service users have of the care they receive from nurses, midwives and other allied professions. Ackerman (1997, in Iles and Sutherland, 2001) identified three types of change: developmental, transitional and transformational. In the first type of developmental change, mentors may be involved because it is planned and tends to focus on the improvement of a skill or process. Some mentors have attended a nursing-specific study day or conference and now have suggestions on how to improve an aspect of nursing care delivery within their own practice area. However, some aspects of change are not quite so linear and do involve a review of the overall service provision. According to Ackerman (1997), transitional change is episodic, planned, second order or may even be radical.

A number of literature sources highlight that transitional change has its foundation in work proposed by Lewin (1951) who described three actions:

1   Unfreezing the existing equilibrium.
2   Moving to a new position.
3   Refreezing in a new equilibrium position (Iles and Sutherland, 2001; Menix, 2003).

Therefore, implementing an aspect of change in the NHS may relate to Lewin's tripartite approach although the effectiveness of implementing change is not without its inherent complexities. Although healthcare may be viewed as a combination of proactive and innovative nursing, midwifery and allied professions, there are nevertheless healthcare professionals who feel that too much change leads to instability and question the well-established policies and procedures already in existence. This scepticism is reflected by Maher in Andalo's (2006) article.

In comparison, the third change perspective is the transformational approach which is developmental and emerges from continuously learning, adapting and improving. Furthermore, Ackerman (1997) states in this approach that a new condition may evolve from the chaotic death of an old state. Approaches to mentorship and the assessment of student nurses in the practice placement have changed in the past few years, and from past experience, this is the new era of the outcomes and proficiencies (NMC, 2004c) and the essential skills clusters assessments (NMC, 2007a). Consider your responses to Mentor Activity 9.2 and compare them with Ackerman's concept.

However, implementing change in the NHS is not without its associated challenges. Taylor (2007) clearly highlights that effective leadership skills are an essential component in ensuring that good healthcare is delivered. She continues to claim that some healthcare personnel must be adaptable enough to manage teams across different professional, clinical and organizational boundaries. Sometimes in order to implement an aspect of change, leadership skills need to conform to the 'three Ps' identified by Hartley and Aimson (2002): the person, the position and the process. Although these three dimensions are significant in influencing the quality of leadership, implementing change does raise other aspects for consideration.

Iles and Sutherland (2001) emphasize that implementing a change into the NHS may incur challenges from the following:

- changing pressures in the environment;
- changing technologies available;
- complex organizations in which individuals and teams are interdependent.

Interprofessional care delivery involving midwives, nurses, and other allied professions relies on a multi-disciplinary team approach. Implementing change by any one of these healthcare professionals may have an impact on the others involved in the patient's journey.

The challenges identified by Iles and Sutherland (2001), Tomey (2004) and Marquis and Huston (2006) are thought-provoking and have inherent warning devices. They certainly warn that within some healthcare organizations that the cause and effect relationships may not be easily apparent and the outcomes may not always be anticipated or, even worse, desirable. Therefore, effective communication and interpersonal skills as identified in the Stage One mentor outcomes will be needed to enhance the change process. Before starting any aspect of change, Iles and Sutherland (2001) advocate that a starting point may be undertaking a SWOT analysis. Reflect back on your responses identified in Mentor Activity 9.2.

An aspect of change needs to be explored and its contribution to improving healthcare exposed. A SWOT analysis helps advocators of any change to justify why they think there is a need for change. SWOT is an acronym for examining the strengths, weaknesses, opportunities and threats of introducing any aspect of change. It is a starting point to convince other team members that the various options, positive and negative indicators, have been considered. The strengths and weaknesses help to clarify the consequences of any change and hopefully, establish the potential positive impact of the action rather than any aspects that would be detrimental and therefore be viewed as negative weaknesses.

'The importance of quality health care cannot be over-emphasized as quality ties into every aspect that health care organizations stand for' (Thorsteinsson, 2002: 32). Throughout the eight domains of mentorship, the NMC (2008a) makes several references to exploring and improving the learning environment for healthcare students so that they are exposed to the delivery of quality healthcare and encouraging mentors to ensure that they have mentorship currency – updated information.

Now read Case study 9.1 and appreciate the importance to the mentor of ensuring that their knowledge is current both as regards their own clinical expertise as well as academic and curriculum changes. The student identified how positive and supportive the mentor had been. Mentorship is challenging and at times students do present the mentor with some areas of concerns. What is important is for the mentor to ensure that their knowledge is up to date in order to maintain their credibility. Whilst working with a third-year student the mentor has the opportunity to share their knowledge of leadership and management, in order to prepare the student for their interviews when applying for their first job as a qualified nurse or midwife. This is a particularly stressful time for the student as they are completing the final requirements in preparation for becoming fit for practice at the point of registration.

As you read Case study 9.1, reflect on your own experiences and the support that you have given to students in your professional career.

CASE STUDY 9.1

A third-year management student had almost completed her final placement and presented her documentation for final verification that she had achieved all the required proficiencies at the required academic level. During this final semester the student must work as an Assistant to the First Level Nurse and consequently must achieve all the identified proficiencies at this advanced level in order to verify that they are Fit for Practice, Fit for Purpose and 'Fit for Registration'.

She discussed with her mentor her achievements both personally and professionally. The student felt that the mentor had supported her throughout her management experience and encouraged her to develop an awareness of some of the management skills that she will need on gaining her registration. The mentor had helped her to develop her confidence dealing with the medical and other allied professions involved in the patient's healthcare experience.

She had discussed the different approaches to leadership, highlighting that she personally favoured a more democratic approach which would encourage all staff members to be involved in management decisions. She knew that she would have to become more assertive. The mentor had reassured her that these skills would develop following registration.

In the preparation for her first job interview, the mentor had spent some time discussing some of the current healthcare issues, policies and procedures that she thought the student needed to read around. The mentor had also spent some time in a mock interview setting which the student thought was very valuable.

For this student, the mentor had worked, guided and supported her throughout this placement but also helped her to capitalize on what she had surreptitiously learnt throughout her training.

Can you apply the same positive approach to your student?

Leadership skills are involved in the following:

- mentor preparation courses
- annual mentor updates
- triennial reviews
- sign–off mentorship.

Mentor preparation programmes

The NMC (2008a: 29) has specified what constitutes an appropriate mentor preparation programme and as from September 2007 these courses must be validated to ensure that they are meeting the recommended guidelines. The basic requirements include:

- A minimum of 10 days, five of which must be protected time for learning.
- Five days are university based and examine associated theory perspectives related to the eight domains of mentorship. There are a number of group activities that encourage discussion of past experiences or future concerns.

- Five days are based in the practice setting undertaking relevant work-based learning activities, preferably under the guidance of an experienced mentor. These activities encourage further discussions in the practice setting and collectively prepare the mentor for their role.
- The combination of theory and practice will help prepare the mentor for their fundamental roles and responsibilities associated with mentorship, as well as providing the opportunity to explore related research findings.
- The course is usually completed in 12 weeks.
- The course may also be linked to post-registration degree pathways allowing mentors to submit an assignment and gain academic credits as well as preparing them for their mentorship role.

Annual mentor updates

Following a mentor preparation course, all mentors are required to attend some form of annual mentor update so that they can keep their knowledge current in order to be aware of the changes in practice and education. There is subsequently a need for all mentors to ensure that their mentorship knowledge is up to date and this can be achieved in a number of ways:

- Mentors should have current knowledge of NMC approved programmes.
- Mentors are given the opportunity to discuss the significant NMC changes to mentorship requirements.
- Mentors are provided with the opportunity to discuss issues associated with their changing role, assessment concerns and ensuring the student is fit for practice, purpose and registration.

Mentor updates are ideally face to face, although other strategies are available – workbooks and e-learning programmes – providing that at least once in three years there is a face-to-face meeting with a university lecturer to ensure that they have the opportunity for discussion of their experiences and concerns with other mentors. Now read Case study 9.2 based on a student's behaviour that concerned a number of mentors and was discussed at a mentor update session.

CASE STUDY 9.2

You have a third-year student nurse who you are concerned about. She always appears to be at the Nurses' Station, and has to be told what to do all the time. You believe she lacks interest in your nursing speciality, although when you tell her of your concerns, she denies this and is adamant that she is progressing well.

She believes that she only has to undertake a task once, in order to achieve her proficiencies. She is upset when you tell her that she is not achieving the level of proficiency that you would expect from a student in their final year.

Your colleagues also share your concerns because when you are not there, the student appears to keep 'disappearing' and not working as a member of the team. This has caused some irritation to your colleagues as the ward is busy and they haven't the time to keep 'chasing' this student to find out what she is doing.

How would you deal with this situation?

Possible areas for consideration:

1   The mentor needs to use their leadership skills in both facilitating learning and assessment in order to manage this situation appropriately.
2   The tripartite approach to undertaking the interviews must be executed and the generated discussion documented to help the student learn and the mentor to develop their skills of managing challenging situations.
3   It is important for the mentor to discuss with the student how they think they are progressing, what proficiencies have and are yet to be achieved. It would be useful to arrange a date and time with the student so that the mentor can review the quality and range of evidence collated.
4   At the designated time, it would be appropriate to arrange a quiet room without any disturbances to allow for a friendly environment to promote discussion.
5   It is important for the mentor to discuss with the student their concerns and those of other staff members, although this must be delivered in a sensitive manner.
6   The aim of the discussion is to discuss with the student the mentor's concerns, the behaviour expected and ultimately to produce an action plan as a positive way forward.

This situation was not managed in this way and the student was very distressed, particularly when the mentor asked if she wanted her to contact her Personal Tutor. The student felt that the situation was becoming distorted and being made worse than it really was. Unfortunately, the way it should have been managed was not the best way so there were lessons to be learnt. This type of case study is thought-provoking and does generate discussions at the mentor update sessions.

Whatever approach is adopted at a mentor update, placement providers will examine the evidence that the mentor has updated their knowledge as an integrated requirement of their triennial review.

The triennial review

Within the recent NMC (2008a) Standards to support learning and assessment in practice are the guidelines that emphasize the importance of the triennial review of mentors. In order for a mentor to maintain their mentor status they have:

- To be registered on the local databases of mentors that is now maintained by service providers.
- To provide evidence that they have mentored at least two students within a three-year period – the way that this is recorded is a local Trust decision.
- To ensure that they attend an annual mentor update.
- To explore and discuss their experiences of assessing in practice as a group activity.
- To plan their ongoing mentor development by meeting the most recent NMC standards for learning and assessing in practice.
- To meet the requirements specified by service providers in order to remain on the database.

The one aspect that concerns mentors is meeting the requirement of mentoring two students in a three-year period. In response, mentors have been advised that their valued contribution to the mentorship team, as the Stage Two mentor or the associate/co-mentor, will ensure that they have currency regarding assessments and completion of the student's documentation. In future, the role will be more accessible if they can contribute to the preparation or undertaking the assessments associated with the essential skills clusters.

Some universities will issue some form of triennial review documentation, which has a record of the types of mentor updates, the actual dates attended as well as confirming the number of students that have been mentored in the three-year time span. This documentation will then be maintained in the NHS Knowledge and Skills Framework Portfolio (DH, 2004) or the Personal Professional Profile as stated in *The Prep Handbook* (NMC, 2008e). This will be discussed every three years as part of an independent professional review or equivalent that is undertaken by the mentor's manager or employer. Timmins (2008: 1) describes a portfolio as 'a collection and cohesive account of work-based learning that contains relevant evidence from practice and a critical reflection on this evidence'. This correlates to the portfolio that is required both pre- and post-registration.

Sign-off mentorship

The sign-off mentor is the term given to the mentor who will be assessing the student on their final placement. There is a debate that mentors who currently are involved in mentoring of management/final placement students have already gained the experience required in order to undertake this role. They are already contributing to the decision that the student is eligible for registration as they are assessing their practice proficiencies at the Assistant to First Level Nurse or Practice Level Four (Bondy, 1988) status. The sign-off mentor will inform the Branch Programme Leader if the student has failed to achieve the appropriate proficiency so that subsequent action can be taken.

The sign-off mentor has to have met additional criteria as stated by the NMC (2008a). The nurse or midwife who is making this ultimate decision regarding the student nurse or midwife's progress must ensure that they are on the same part or sub-part of the register that the student is intending to be registered on. The specific criteria include the following:

- placement providers must ensure that a nurse or midwife designated as a sign-off mentor is:
  - identified on the local register as a sign-off mentor, they are annotated on the database;
  - registered on the same part of the register;
  - working in the same field of practice as that in which the student intends to qualify.

In addition, the sign-off mentor must have:

- clinical currency and capability in the field in which the student is being assessed;
- a working knowledge of current programme requirements, practice assessment strategies and relevant changes in education and practice for the student they are assessing;
- an understanding of the NMC registration requirements and the contribution they make to the achievement of these requirements;
- an in-depth understanding of their accountability to the NMC for the decision they must make to pass or fail a student when assessing proficiency requirements at the end of a programme;
- been supervised on at least three occasions for signing off proficiency by an existing sign-off mentor;
- a working knowledge of current programme requirements, practice assessment strategies and relevant changes in education and practice for the student they are assessing.
- achieved these requirements;
- an understanding of the NMC registration requirements and the contribution they make to meeting these requirements;
- an in-depth understanding of their accountability to the NMC for the decision they make to pass or fail a student when assessing proficiency requirements at the end of a programme. (NMC, 2008a: 21)

The requirements of the sign-off mentor and the importance of that accountability are or will be a focus topic at mentor updates throughout 2009 in some universities. The sign-off mentor role started with all student nurses undertaking pre-registration training as from September 2007. They will spend the required 40 per cent of time with their mentor and an additional one hour per week protected time (NMC, 2008a: 31) in order that the mentor can discuss the student's progress, monitor the construction of the Student's Portfolio and examine their Ongoing Achievement Record. This record is a collection of all the student's final interviews throughout their training, identifying their strengths, weaknesses, and if any action plans have been implemented in order to meet any identified deficits or unsafe practices. The sign-off mentor must have access to this complete record in order to assist them make their final decision of the student's suitability for entry to the register.

All midwifery students can only be supported and assessed by sign-off mentors who have met the additional sign-off criteria. From September 2007, all students on pre-registration midwifery programmes must follow these requirements.

The NMC (2008a: 33) highlights the importance of *due regard* which means that the sign-off mentor must be a registered nurse who has their name on the same part of the register that coincides with the branch training programme completed by the student. Similarly, only a registered midwife is allowed to sign off a midwifery student.

This chapter has explored the associated theoretical concepts associated with the skills and process of effective leadership skills. There is value in appreciating the different leadership styles and how they have an impact on team cohesion and development. Teams do vary and change according to the sociology of nursing and the ever changing nursing culture, changes in ward or departmental leader, staff promotions, staff terminating their contracts or moving to other healthcare settings which can result in changes to team dynamics. The NMC (2008a) introduced their vision of mentorship now and in the future. The changes to the standards for mentorship have been implemented in mentor preparation courses and mentor update sessions have been subsequently amended to meet those requirements. The frequently asked questions are often a reflection of mentors' and students' concerns to changes that are currently or intend to be implemented.

Frequently asked questions

Mentors

Q. I find it difficult to ensure that I spend enough time mentoring the student that I am supposed to. How am I to ensure that I fulfil the requirements of the sign-off mentor?

A. This is a question that is frequently asked at mentor updates. It is anticipated that you ensure that your mentorship approach follows the principles of continuous assessment. Therefore, on a weekly or fortnightly basis you will be reviewing the student's progress and offering suggestions if there are any areas of weakness. There is a commitment that there should be one hour protected time in order that the mentor can read previous mentor's comments and which action plans were recommended and implemented. The problem of the ongoing achievement record is that the sign-off mentor will have to rely on all the previous mentors undertaking their role with equal commitment. However, the sign-off mentor is predominantly assessing against the level that the student is currently at.

Q. How can I guarantee to have the protected one hour per week with the student if I am going to be their sign-off mentor?

A. The concept of the sign-off mentor was introduced by the NMC in 2006 and managers and those involved as service providers were made aware of this requirement. There has to be an agreement that the sign-off mentor does have this protected time in order that the practice placement honours their agreement as part of the student's final semester training. At mentor updates this is a frequently asked question and the response from those present is a sceptical one indicating that there is doubt that this time will be allowed. The mentor will need to show their manager the NMC (2008a) mentor standards requirements and discuss their concerns.

Students

Q. On my last day on placement my mentor was very busy so he wanted me to leave my Ongoing Achievement Record with him to sign and he said he would send it on to me. I was told by my Tutor that we were not to do this but when I explained this to him he became annoyed with me. Did I do the right thing?

A. The Ongoing Achievement Record is the student's responsibility and they must ensure that it does not get lost. All students need to think carefully before leaving their document anywhere because they must present this to their sign-off mentor on their final placement, in their final year, as a complete record of their training and in order to successfully complete their practice assessments for their nurse training programme.

Q. I am concerned that my mentor will not have time to complete my essential skills clusters assessment because the ward is so busy, according to a student who has just been on that placement. What will happen if this occurs?

(Continued)

(Continued)

A. All students must now stress at their initial/preliminary interview what their learning outcomes for that placement are. As part of that discussion you must discuss the assessment, gain advice on how you can prepare and develop the skills to be assessed. At the intermediate interview, the student's progress will be reviewed and a potential date set for the assessment. The student can then work with the practice placement team, following the criteria that they will be assessed against, in order to ensure that they are adequately prepared. Any concerns you must discuss with your mentor.

Chapter summary

This chapter has focused on the process of leadership and how it is an integrated role within mentorship. Having completed this chapter you have learned about:

- the importance of leadership within the profession of nursing starting with the healthcare student through to fulfilling the outcomes within domain eight of the mentor standards;
- the need to have a plan of the healthcare student's experience during their practice placement in order that they can strive to achieve the optimum within their professional development in that area;
- the need to be aware of leadership styles, to review your manager's own approach and how it may have an impact on the healthcare student's practice experience;
- the need to implement and manage change within contemporary healthcare in order to deliver the most effective care for patients and service users;
- the need for annual mentor updates and to ensure that the mentor's knowledge reflects current approaches and practices within mentorship.

Further reading

Jones, L. (2008) 'Leadership in the "new" NHS', *Nursing Management*, 15(6): 32–5.

This is a really interesting and thought-provoking article that explores the importance of leadership as part of a nurse's role. The article is linked to both the Royal College of Nursing and the Open University and reviews the way forward if nurses wish to develop their leadership skills.

10

The mentors' experiences of mentorship

David Kinnell

Introduction

Throughout the different chapters of this book the intention has been to explore the expanding role and responsibilities of the mentor within contemporary healthcare, whether working with nursing or healthcare students. The predominant feature throughout has been the exploration of the eight domains of mentorship and their associated outcomes pertinent to both Stage One: for all nurses and midwives and Stage Two: mentors (NMC, 2008a). Wherever appropriate, this has been discussed and compared with some of the inherent complexities of mentorship that have evolved as the process of assessment and accountability has become more established. The mentor activities, case studies and frequently asked questions have been incorporated in order to enhance the mentors' understanding of mentorship that is appropriate for newly qualified staff during their first year of registration, for mentors undertaking formal mentor training or for existing mentors as part of their annual update. Throughout this final chapter, the focus will be on mentorship experiences of those mentors who are actually involved in supporting students in contemporary healthcare.

The experience of mentorship – the mentors' perspective

To summarize your conception of mentorship, reflect on your experiences since completing your Stage Two: mentor training and discuss the question in Mentor Activity 10.1.

MENTOR ACTIVITY 10.1

What has becoming a mentor meant to you as a person and as a nurse?
Reflect on this question before continuing with this chapter.

This discussion could generate richer and more meaningful subjective data that emphasizes your perception of your role change and the ongoing development of professional responsibilities within contemporary healthcare. During their yearly updates, mentors explore the above question and often the response relates to the realization that the extent of the roles and responsibilities of mentorship seem to be an ever changing process influenced by amendments in the student nurse training programme. This subjective evaluative awareness also highlights the quality and the personal professional fulfilment of the relationship between the mentor and the student within an ever changing healthcare environment. However, this question may highlight areas of further development as mentors share the discussion of their mentorship experiences.

The question in Mentor Activity 10.1 was also the actual research question used in a small study involving eight mentors from different adult branch nursing specialities (Kinnell, 2004). Throughout this chapter the qualitative data gained will be examined and contrasted with other research findings. This chapter is not a critique of the research methods, methodology, reliability or validity adopted whilst undertaking this research but is used to value the qualitative findings revealed by the mentors' discussions which have since been used both in subsequent mentor preparation programmes and yearly mentor updates. Therefore, it will be useful for mentors to contrast their mentorship experiences with those discussed by the eight mentors involved and subsequently differentiate between idealism and reality. Some of the eight mentors commented that it is very difficult sometimes to balance their responsibilities between their role as a qualified nurse, managing wards and departments, and that of providing quality mentorship support.

The research study involved undertaking a one-to-one, face-to-face interview with qualified Registered Nurses in order to gather research data that would describe the mentor's personal experiences and how they responded and adapted to the increasing demands. These qualified nurses undertake the role of a mentor, in various acute and critical healthcare settings within three different hospitals. Morton-Cooper and Palmer (2000: 39) state: 'Mentoring is dynamic and exciting, in part because of its kaleidoscopic nature and also because it is a relatively complex concept, made more intricate by the various connotations placed on it.' They emphasize that the process can be open to interpretation and can be adapted to meet the needs of a number of different settings. Therefore, because of its diversity in application, mentorship can be used to the benefit of those parties involved, although to be successful, both the mentor and student have to appreciate the potential that the role involves.

Pulsford, Boit and Owen (2002) in their research devised and distributed a questionnaire that sought to gain both quantitative and qualitative data. The questionnaire was sent to four hundred mentors and the one qualitative question asked, 'What would make your role as a mentor easier and or more fulfilling?' In response, Pulsford et al. identified a number of 'Factors that would enhance mentors' ability to provide practice-based learning for student nurses'. The responses included the following themes:

1   *Time for undertaking mentoring role.* A large number of respondents reported problems with finding time to spend with students. Several would prefer supernumerary time, or additional staff cover to allow them to spend more time with students.
2   *Management support.* This included guidance as to how to prioritize mentoring students, in relation to other professional demands placed on practitioners
3   *Partnership with the HEI.* Respondents wanted more information from the higher education institutions about students' placements, and in particular, more feedback as to students' progress.
4   *Practice learning documentation.* There was a desire for less paperwork, or more 'user-friendly' documents.
5   *More appropriate use of placements.* Respondents wanted students to come for longer placements. The results highlighted that more thought should be given to the nature of the placement area when allocating students and a more even throughput of students.
6   *Students' motivation.* There were a few comments about students' commitment and motivation, with respondents feeling that some students needed to be more motivated.
7   *Extra pay.* A small number identified that extra responsibility needed some financial reward.

There are a number of other research studies that have tried to understand the reality of being a mentor as well as juggling all their other roles and responsibilities. My study involving the eight mentors focused on their subjective experiences of mentoring. The qualitative approach adopted related to phenomenology that encourages participants to share their world with the researcher. This is in marked contrast to a quantitative research method that is interested in statistical data. The value of phenomenology is that it allows the researcher to study the identified phenomena in depth, and not merely engage in superficial analysis as pertinent to some other research methods. The eight mentors said that they were all willing to discuss their experiences of the 'reality' of being a mentor.

The eight mentors represented Accident and Emergency (one), Care of the Older Person (one), Critical Care (two), General Medicine (two), and General Surgery (two). These included areas of my own nursing background having worked as a Staff Nurse in Accident and Emergency, Critical Care and General Surgery, as well as a Charge Nurse in Accident and Emergency, General Surgery and as an Agency Nurse in Care of the Older Person, in a number of nursing homes. The advantage of this group was the ability to share a professional commonality. Hence, this was appropriate for sharing the being-in-the-world approach advocated with Heideggerian hermeneutic phenomenology (Corben, 1999; Hallett, 1995; Koch, 1999). The taped interviews were unstructured, lasted from 45 minutes to one hour, and all started with the same question as stated in Mentor Activity 10.1. The progression was dependent on spontaneous exploration of the mentors' responses and the contributions helped in the creation of new knowledge that may be used in the future (Holloway and Fulbrook, 2001).

In order to ensure that the hermeneutic phenomenological approach is effective, it is important to ensure that the interview progresses by showing reciprocal interest in what the participant is saying, and to use sensitive probing to ascertain the individual's cognitive and humanistic functioning (Clarke, 2006). This is an attempt to understand the person's self-concept, with particular emphasis on self-efficacy, highlighting the effectiveness of undertaking the mentor's role. Heidegger's concept of 'what it is to be human' offers a contribution to exploring the intricacies and complexities of mentorship. The interview can be regarded as a valuable data gathering tool, as it allows the researcher to obtain information regarding, 'the participants' personal characteristics, experiences, values, attitudes and behaviours' (Harris and Inayatt, 1997: 73). This is supported by Burnard (2005) and McCann and Clark (2005). The eight mentors shared their mentorship expectations and aspirations and how they were faced with a dilemma. Some of them had to appreciate the dichotomy between what they wanted to do (facilitate and assess learning in the practice setting) and what they had to do, manage a hospital ward or department. All the discourse was recorded on tape. During the transcribing of the tape recordings, the frustrations in the tone of their voices and the paralinguistic emphasis that some mentors did express when faced with this dichotomy were evident. Complete Mentor Activity 10.2 before reading the research findings.

MENTOR ACTIVITY 10.2

What are some of the frustrations that mentors feel when trying to balance what they should do with what they would like to do, when mentoring a student?

Consider this question and make a note of the main areas of your concern before continuing this chapter.

Taylor (1995) explores the conceptual issue of 'the nature of phenomenon' and in her article explains the interpretations pertinent to phenomenology in nursing research. She specifies that the phenomenon actually begins with the people involved, in their place and time, and is subsequently a reflection of 'the nature of people as human beings, who find themselves within the context of a healthcare institution, who are living and making sense of their experiences' (ibid.: 76). During the data analysis this statement was significant as it allowed the opportunity to examine the mentors' descriptions of their experiences and the difference between idealism and reality. A predominant concern expressed was the frustration of wanting to be an effective role model and ensure that the practice setting was conducive for learning (Bahn, 2001; Kopp, 2001; Quinn and Hughes, 2007).

'What has becoming a mentor meant to you as a person and as a nurse?'

As part of the data analysis it was evident that there were a number of responses that were similar, these were grouped together as a number of resultant constituent clusters (Spencer, 2007) which were then categorized in the resultant structure of eight key elements, six of which will be explored throughout this chapter (Table 10.1).

1 Achieving acceptability

Most of the eight mentors highlighted the significance of helping to make the student nurse feel valued, that they belonged, were respected and needed. In response, it was anticipated that the student nurse would view the mentor as helpful and this would influence how effective the mentor felt they were undertaking their mentorship role. The role of the mentor also meant that because they were working on a one-to-one basis that they

TABLE 10.1   *Elements and their constituent clusters generated from the research data*

Elements	Constituent clusters
1 Achieving acceptability	Need to be valued
	Help to feel they belong
	Respected and needed
	Part of a team
	Let them find their feet
	Talk about what is expected
	Introduce to other staff
	Help to interact
2 Achievement	Help to realize progress made
	Developing clinical skills
	Meeting expectations
	Getting through student's paperwork
	Meeting the grade
	Identifying actual problems
	Don't stand over them
	Consensus assessment
3 Commitment	Sharing personal experiences
	Readiness to teach
	Should spend more time
	Challenged
	Interested in education
4 Creating an effective learning environment	Maintaining up-to-date knowledge/skills
	Develop critical thinking approach
	Resources
	Different teaching strategies
	Supportive team
	Teaching on the ward
	Using time effectively
	Multi-disciplinary team approach
5 Responsibility	Personally responsible
	Student-centred
	Practice-centred
	Impinge on job
	Asking questions
	Extra pressure
	Change in role
6 Self-efficacy	Attitudes
	Feelings and emotions
	Perceptions
	Self-concept
	Self-ideal discrepancy
	Disharmony

should help the student nurse feel part of the team as stated in domain one (NMC, 2008a). Being accepted by the student nurse established a personal sense of achievement by the mentor. It helped them to feel that what they did for the student was appreciated. However, there were concerns regarding the most appropriate way of establishing positive feelings about being accepted. The mentors discussed what they did to help, particularly during the student's initial induction into the ward or department (RCN, 2007b).

> I like to make them feel that they have become part of the team and their job is just as important as somebody else's. (mentor: Accident and Emergency)

> I try to introduce them to any staff members that they come across, like the doctors, introduce them to them, this is so and so … I make sure that the patients know that they are new so that they don't expect too much of them. (mentor: General Surgery)

The eight mentors explained that they tried to adopt an individualistic approach. Allowing the student time to 'find their feet' and talking about what was expected were two common approaches identified. Some mentors felt they should be there on the student's first day in order to introduce them to other staff, the patients and help reduce any feelings of anxiety. Reviewing how effective this process had worked for them, some mentors identified that the majority of students had appreciated their efforts and that they had established a firm basis for the rest of their allocation. The RCN (2007b: 45) states: 'As a mentor you are required to offer the student support and guidance in the practice area.' The mentors emphasized how important it was for them to establish a welcoming approach so that the student felt that they belonged, and in most cases this had worked well.

According to Gross (2005) and Hayes (2005), the need to feel valued and gaining a sense of belonging is identified by Maslow (1954) in his classic theory 'hierarchy of human needs'. Once the student has been accepted, and they feel respected and needed as part of the team, they can progress, according to Maslow, and develop their self-esteem, i.e. how good they feel about themselves. Assisting the student during their progression had given the mentor a sense of achievement, and all eight stated that they felt instrumental in accomplishing a sense of positive attainment. This had resulted in them acquiring a 'good' reputation of being an 'effective' mentor, which was recognition that was acknowledged by students being allocated to their practice setting. This acknowledgement of their efforts and commitment to mentorship had established a personal sense of worth, knowing that they were fulfilling the expectations inherent within the mentor's role.

Indeed, undertaking an unrealistic assessment too soon would not have enhanced the mentor's reputation and hence their own view of their acceptability to the student and the placement philosophy. One mentor (General Medicine) reflected on her own student nurse training and stated:

Thinking about it – going on some placements, some of the trained staff just did not want to know ... You know, you might as well have been that curtain ... they did not want to teach you ... they don't want you in their environment.

However, this was not the impression of all the eight mentors. In contrast, one mentor (Critical Care Unit) emphasized that the experience she had shared with her first student nurse was extremely positive. She said, 'That night I enjoyed her company thoroughly. I did because, possibly because of the rapport initially, had I been threatening ... or patronising, possibly she would have looked fed up being with me.' She continued, 'She wanted to be with me. I felt valued but she didn't make me feel like she was my shadow, that she did not ... and I was getting positive feedback.' Hurley and Snowden (2008) explored the role of mentoring within critical care settings and examined mentoring in times of change.

Listening to the tape recordings and re-reading the transcripts from all eight participants, my interpretation is that the mentors wanted to prove to themselves that they had achieved a sense of acceptance and recognition from the student nurses. They acknowledged that their role was continually expanding according to local healthcare needs but being accepted as an 'effective' mentor was an achievement they personally wanted. Some of them made exceptional efforts to ensure that they were accepted by the student and as part of the mentoring team on their ward or department.

'During the initial interview with the student if there is anything that they want to learn about, then one of us will put together a package and will do a presentation and talk for them' (mentor: General Medicine). She continued to identify how she had changed whilst becoming a mentor and how she still feels if the students make negative comments to their Personal Tutor in the School of Nursing, without having first discussed them on the ward.

Another mentor summarized her viewpoint:

In A and E we are a very close team, we just share ideas amongst ourselves. We work together to support the student and help them feel that they belong. I say to them if you feel that I am asking you to do something that you are not quite prepared to do, you must tell me.

She continued to emphasize that for mentorship to work, the student must trust the mentor, and vice versa. Therefore, in order to gain acceptance, the mentors highlighted how they hoped that they achieved a very open and friendly rapport and this would enhance the relationship between the two.

It is inevitable that part of their role does relate to the process of assessment and this is the second element of 'achievement' that was identified when examining the commonality within the qualitative data generated and summarizes the constituent clusters, comments common to all eight mentors (see Box 10.1).

Box 10.1   Element One – Achieving acceptability

Reflect on the mentor's comments and consider how pertinent they are to your experiences of mentorship.

---

2 Achievement

According to the eight mentors, the transition to becoming a mentor entailed acquiring responsibility for the assessment process and how they individually contributed to that process. This responsibility was viewed by many mentors as integral to mentoring. By assessing the student nurse's competency achievements, it helped them realize their progress. This helped the mentors to identify their own development of clinical skills and the extent of meeting expectations on both parts. This encouraged them to review their own personal achievements of participating in a process that was initially viewed by some of them as daunting. Developing their skills of completing the documentation and having to make a judgement about their student nurse's practical competency was an achievement for all eight mentors and related effectively to the domain three outcomes (NMC, 2008a).

It did become difficult for some of them when they had to decide if the student nurse was actually meeting the grade according to their level of training and they had to make a judgement that would influence that individual's progress. There was a consensus of concern expressed by the mentors regarding how they would deal with problematic students, perhaps one of the most demanding decisions of their role (Duffy, 2004; Duffy and Hardicre, 2007a). Some of them reflected on experiences so far, stating that it was not helpful to stand over the student constantly watching every move. If there was any doubt in their assessment, the mentors stated that they did rely on a consensus approach, gaining the opinions of their colleagues, to ensure an objective assessment. This involved colleagues working with the student in practice and feeding back to them as the identified mentor how successful the learning outcomes or proficiencies had been achieved (NMC, 2004c).

Helping students to complete their Student Portfolio of Evidence (NMC, 2004c: 34) and understanding the differences in the range of evidence had caused some of the mentors some apprehension and concern because of the lack of personal experience in portfolio construction. Being able to confidently sign the verification statement that their student had achieved all the placement outcomes or proficiencies in association with the range of evidence presented was a skill that mentors have to achieve when first undertaking the role. Many of them reflected on how effective they were attaining this achievement and how they felt once their confidence had been established.

The sense of achievement was also influenced by how well they were able to implement the cardinal criteria of assessment (Quinn and Hughes, 2007). This cognitive checklist had helped the mentors to ascertain if they were achieving validity and reliability in their assessments, as well as considering the practicality and the impact of discriminatory power. In order to feel that they were developing the skills of assessment, being able to compare and integrate Rowntree's (1997) model with the cardinal criteria, had been an achievement that all mentors stated they had and were continuing to develop. 'I think I needed the Mentor Training Course to be taught how to assess because it was something that I'd not really done before' (mentor: Critical Care Unit).

One of the mentors from General Surgery highlighted how she felt that she was achieving what was expected of her.

> I've been involved with students as much as I can and getting feedback … assessing what she does … but I still find it, she just doesn't do things right … but nothing major. I'm still finding it a little difficult to give feedback because it can be a bit awkward.

Each mentor identified that they needed to be objective and avoid any aspect of subjectivity when it came to completing the student nurse's documentation. They had to decide whether the student had achieved the stated outcome in association with their level of training – yes or no. Once they had made their decision, they recorded it in the appropriate place. What the mentors also agreed with was the influence of assessment bias. Whilst assessing students there is a temptation to overrate them (halo effect) in terms of their popularity on the placement. Alternatively, it is possible to underrate them (horn effect), if they were a shy, introverted student nurse. In either situation, there was an element of subjectivity that at times was difficult to deal with.

The competencies that student nurses have to achieve are based on criterion referencing (Quinn and Hughes, 2007). This approach is more objective and should be based on a more unbiased effective assessment. However, some mentors discussed how having this knowledge and understanding was helpful, nevertheless they felt it was sometimes difficult to achieve effectively. They felt that they had developed and one of their main achievements was utilizing the skill of being objective.

Two of the mentors had been involved in supporting one of their colleagues with a problematic student, by contributing to a group consensus report. They had been asked to provide statements of competency which they felt was awkward but nevertheless highlighted the impact of discriminatory power. 'As it happens, it was all of us that were finding the same problem and needed to highlight it … and it was dealt with' (mentor: General Medicine).

However, when dealing with a problematic student nurse, one mentor (General Surgery) reflected on the experience and stated:

> If we are not happy with someone, it's our responsibility to speak up and say so and that's quite frightening … You do realise that at the end of the day we are the ones that are saying to you 'why has this person qualified?'

The mentors found that their transition into the mentor's role was a positive achievement, relating theory to their experiences in practice had been a positive experience for each one of them.

However, there were so many other issues identified and these have been clustered to form the next element: commitment, but before reading that section, complete Mentor Activity 10.3.

MENTOR ACTIVITY 10.3

How do the feelings of the eight mentors explored throughout this element of achievement mirror your experiences of mentorship?

Consider this question before reading the next section.

3 Commitment

A number of issues identified by the mentors related to the need to establish and maintain a commitment to facilitating learning in the practice setting, a requirement that relates to domain two (NMC, 2008a). Some mentors discussed the need to share personal experiences of their own student nurse training, having a readiness to teach and spend more time with the student nurse. However, the consensus of opinion was that becoming a mentor was very challenging and being interested in education was an essential prerequisite. The mentors all identified that trying to show commitment and fulfil all the other roles and responsibilities expected of them as a team member and mentor was problematic.

They all highlighted how they had made an attempt to meet those expectations. Some mentors felt that sharing their personal experiences and trying to spend as much time as possible with the student, was a positive commitment. Although the specified requirement is that a student should spend at least 40% of their time with a mentor (NMC, 2008a), these eight mentors wanted to show more of a commitment. Lloyd Jones et al. (2001) identified that student nurses spending time with their mentors was essential in helping them to learn technical skills as well as interpersonal and professional skills central to nursing. This could help resolve some of the students' concerns identified by Higginson (2006). This is a constituent feature that is supported by Koh (2002) and appeared as an aspect of the mentor's role that was highlighted by each of the eight mentors.

> I should have spent more time ... with the student role and the mentor role rather than the business of the ward ... You just have to juggle and prioritize everything all the time ... but you try and put students on your higher priority ... but it is very difficult when you are so busy. (mentor: General Medicine)

However, there was a general consensus from all eight mentors that trying to involve the student nurse in some form of learning or activity was representative of their commitment to becoming a mentor. Watson (1999: 259) states, 'Mentors felt that they offer clinical support to students and facilitated their learning while acting as role models for them.' So there was an agreement among the eight mentors that although maintaining commitment to the mentor's role was certainly problematic, it was certainly an aspect of their role that they wanted to maintain, sometimes this was taking it to the extreme. One of them stated that she said to one student, 'It is your responsibility to follow me, I am not going to keep looking over my shoulder ... I'm going to the bathroom ... no, no, you don't have to follow me there' (mentor: Accident and Emergency).

Morton-Cooper and Palmer (2000) as well as Andrews and Chilton (2000) emphasize the importance of showing a positive commitment to mentorship. The mentors stated:

> Mentor's approach must fit with the theory/research ... so as to support the theory and practice relationship. (mentor: Critical Care Unit)

> I need more of an in-depth knowledge for teaching ... so I can put a good argument forward, discuss it more ... pros and cons. (mentor: Accident and Emergency)

To continually attempt to update your own knowledge as well as achieving all the other attributes that are pertinent to the mentor's role was identified by the eight mentors as a strong act of commitment. Many of them stated that they had attended study days in their own time. There was, therefore, a commitment to balance work and private lives accordingly as well as meeting the requirements for the NMC (2008c).

However, although the acquisition of in-depth knowledge enhanced the individual's ability of becoming a mentor, it also helps them to meet the requirements encompassed within *The NHS Knowledge and Skills Framework* (DH, 2004).

Becoming a mentor, acquiring appropriate knowledge and showing a commitment to future developments were attributes that the mentors highlighted that they had already attained or wanted to aspire to in the future. Some mentors stated that they are continuing to use the research-based knowledge examined when undertaking the Mentor Training Programme as they develop their knowledge and skills as mentors.

> It does come back to confidence, self-esteem, obviously because when you've got a student, you know … you need the qualifications to help them with their education, to teach. (mentor: Critical Care Unit)

> It made me change in the way that I think, when I have got students … um, it makes me think, 'Oh yes, they are learning this way', or it made me realise what my qualifications are. (mentor: General Surgery)

Throughout each of the interviews, the mentors emphasized that if they were to be effective in their role, it would mean them showing a commitment to both developing their practical skills and acquiring theory so that they can mentor a student nurse with confidence. Some of the mentors indicated that they felt that having qualifications enabled them to feel knowledgeable, and ahead of the student nurse, in response, the student nurse would acknowledge their expertise, and therefore they would feel good about themselves and re-commit.

The constituent cluster for this element emphasizes the individual themes and topics that the mentors discussed, they were then subsequently grouped or clustered together as having some commonality. The element is the broad perspective word or theme that amalgamates these constituent clusters together in order that their qualitative value can be explored, discussed and analysed. Throughout this element three of the mentors emphasized the reasons why they wanted to show a commitment for further education and subsequently, contribute towards creating an effective learning environment – consider element 3 (see Box 10.2).

Box 10.2   Element Three – Commitment

Reflect on the individual aspects and themes within the constituent cluster and consider their significance for your practice area.

---

4 Creating an effective learning environment

The fourth element was clearly identified by each mentor and they all valued its significance as part of becoming a mentor. Each of the different practice settings has made a concerted attempt to develop and maintain their individual placements as effective learning environments. The mentors stressed that this was reflected in the student nurses' evaluation of their practice experiences. Establishing an environment that is conducive to learning was identified by Kopp (2001), Bahn (2001) and Spouse (2001) as important to success. According to Spouse (2001: 150), 'As novices, students relied very much upon the help of their mentor to guide them. With increasing confidence they became more self-directing and able to gain help with a variety of sources.'

One of the mentors (Critical Care Unit) reflected on her skills and believed they included:

- maintaining and updating her knowledge and skills;
- encouraging student nurses to learn;
- acting as a resource but also recommending further resources as an alternative or to support existing recommended literature.

In some practice settings, the mentor does not always have the influence that they would like to. As identified by some of them, in some practice settings it is difficult to prevent the loss of books and journals. Hopes of establishing an effective resource centre on the ward or department have been dashed for some of them. In one case the mentor stated: 'We have got resources on the ward – flipcharts, overhead projectors but you need a room for the teaching session' (mentor: Care of Older Person).

These were teaching resources that some of the mentors stated they would like to have, although not all of them agreed these were essential in order to create an effective learning environment for the students. Indeed, reflecting on this aspect of the mentor's role, one mentor (General Surgery) stated: 'I think for them to come into the clinical setting they don't want to be taken into the Day Room, in front of a flipchart.' There were different opinions on what constitutes an effective learning environment. She continued, 'I try to get them out with the stoma nurse, endoscopy, whatever … so that they can learn in that way because I can't offer them that.'

Ausubel et al. (1978) identify an 'assimilation theory of meaningful learning' in which they advocate that the most single important factor influencing learning is what the student already knows. They propose that once this is established, then it can be built upon. The mentor needs to be able to identify the student's previous experiences, knowledge, skills, weaknesses and help to develop them accordingly.

The eight mentors all stated that they tried to make the healthcare experience a valued and significant insight into their nursing speciality. Depending on the stage of training and experience of the student nurse, some of their learning objectives were either too vague or too ambitious. The mentors all reflected on their skills of sorting these out, praising the student for their ambitious outlook but establishing realistic and achievable learning outcomes that can be used throughout the allocated placement.

Throughout the interviews, the mentors reflected on their facilitation skills as part of the day-to-day process of mentorship. Although this is described by Morton–Cooper and Palmer (2000), the mentors discussed a collective overview of the reality of their lived experiences so far. This is an important element because Koh (2002: 35) states, 'The shift of focus on education is based on the fundamental belief that nursing is a practice-based profession and that the quality of learning hinges on the quality of clinical experiences.' There was consensus amongst the mentors that they all did their best to contribute to creating and establishing an effective learning environment.

A dichotomy was identified between what the mentors wanted to achieve and what was achievable. Some of them discussed problems they encountered by trying to balance the many roles and responsibilities that they had now acquired, with creating an effective learning environment being only one aspect. Corlett (2000) explored the ongoing debate related to the supposed existence of the 'theory–practice' gap in nurse education. However, all the mentors stressed that this debated concept was not as prevalent as some of the literature seems to indicate (Kitson, 2001; Landers, 2000; Wilson-Barnett et al., 1995).

Some pertinent related comments made by the mentors included: 'It's rewarding because your student goes away and you think that you have had an impact whether little or great, you've had some impact on that student nurse's learning' (mentor: Critical Care Unit). However, according to another, 'Thinking of ways to improve how you are helping your mentored student and your colleagues … even, your junior staff is not always that easy' (mentor: General Medicine). This problem is growing because of the escalating demands placed on the Staff Nurse. 'You know that the student's with you, you are meant to be helping the student and you're not' (mentor: General Surgery).

So, in reality, becoming a mentor is a challenge, it is necessary to use your knowledge and understanding of facilitation skills, to have the pivotal focus of enhancing student involvement in the practice setting. Reflecting on the transition to the mentor's role, some stated that being involved with training the student nurse and identifying ways to improve the experience by encouraging involvement, was paramount to the success of the student's practice placement. Throughout the interviews there was no doubt from the mentor's lived experiences that they had to accept change in their role and absorb the added responsibility of mentoring – hence the next significant element.

5 Responsibility

The role of the mentor does have inherent responsibilities. Many of the mentors referred to a personal responsibility and how they realized the importance of developing both a student-centred and a practice-centred philosophy. The most highlighted change that impinged on their job as a mentor was dealing with student nurses and trying to answer the almost constant flow of questions. Having discussed their experiences, some mentors were adamant that this had caused extra pressure, extra stress on them and that there was certainly a change in their professional role and responsibilities.

This claim was supported by Brennan and Hutt (2001: 181) who stated, 'An increase in the number of learners in the clinical environment, has meant that we have had to look at new and innovative ways to support both learners and Practitioners to ensure that the clinical placement is a positive learning experience.' Each of the mentors identified how there was an increase in the number of students being sent to their practice setting, which meant that they were given more added responsibility. Some of the mentors expressed the impact of the extra responsibility:

> You are particularly responsible and accountable for your student, so anything they do, say, write down, you know that it is your head that is on the block. (mentor: Accident and Emergency)

> Having a student does impinge on your job … it's very difficult, especially within the critical care area where you have got an agenda for your shift and that agenda is coming every five minutes. (mentor: Critical Care Unit)

However, some of the mentors also stressed the need to be realistic and balance the added responsibility accordingly: 'I don't agree working with your mentor all the time' (mentor: Care of the Older Person) who continued by saying: 'It is good to take things from different people, so as a mentor myself and working with students, they need to see different ways.'

No matter how the individual deals with the added responsibility, the necessity of adopting the mentor's role was emphasized by many of the mentors. One mentor (General Surgery) made a poignant comment:

> You also realize how difficult it is for people who are mentors, that if there are only so many on the ward ... there is quite a lot of pressure on you to be a mentor ... So you realize that you are taking a bit of pressure off other people because there is more ... more to go around.

The five general elements examined so far have tried to explore the mentor's role from a number of different perspectives. The next section relates to the human element of the mentor as a person, and how they see that the role has subsequently changed them and their ability to cope but before you read this, complete Mentor Activity 10.4.

MENTOR ACTIVITY 10.4

Consider both elements four and five then reflect on their significance to your practice area.

Then continue with reading the final sixth element.

---

6 Self-efficacy

The constituent cluster highlighted aspects of the mentors' interviews that focused on their individual humanistic qualities and their feelings of how successful they have been at undertaking the role. One area of interest generated during the investigation was to discuss how the eight mentors had changed personally, as well as professionally, by becoming a mentor. Focusing on their thoughts, feelings and how they had changed as a person, a number of the mentors related to changes in their attitudes towards students, the feelings and emotions that this aspect of their job entailed.

For some of them, there was a dichotomy between what their perception of the mentor's role encompassed and successfully undertaking the role. This perceptual distortion had influenced the mentors' own self-concept of themselves as people, their self-ideal discrepancy (difference between who they would like to be and who they really are) and consequently a state of incongruence (Rogers, 1951). This issue relates to how ideally they would like to mentor but in reality they felt they could be more effective. This was discussed by all eight mentors. This sixth element focused upon how the mentors were affected and changed in response to how they viewed the added responsibility. Gross (2005) explains that, according to Bandura (1977), 'self-efficacy' means the extent a person believes they can meet and cope with the new responsibilities. It relates to their responses to how they can meet and develop their potential, being aware of what they can achieve.

The eight mentors identified that there is a difference between being a mentor and being an 'effective' mentor. This is significantly related to how effective the individuals can achieve what they want to achieve, in order to satisfy their perception of what an effective mentor should be. Many of the mentors did reflect on how becoming a mentor had changed them as a person, influencing their attitudes towards the role, and their understanding of what it has meant becoming a mentor. Some of their comments included: 'I looked at mentors as a role model and knowing that suddenly ... I don't really feel that now after eighteen months ... so obviously feel a little bit I'm not good enough in that field' (mentor: General Surgery). She continued by saying,

> I think I am on a bit of a downward trough at the moment because you think about all the questions that you might be asked and you know how much information you're expected to know ... now that you are a mentor and at the moment, I am not really ready for that.

However, in contrast, one mentor (General Medicine) stated: 'I think you identify what qualities you have got, what kind of person you are, you know ... it makes you stop and think ... I think it's being approachable and having the knowledge and the confidence to actually give the same to the students.'

Throughout this chapter the aim has been to examine the mentor's role from the mentor's own perspective. A selection of qualitative data has been identified and explored based on the constituent clusters and six associated elements. The rationale for including this chapter has been to help new Stage One: Nurses and Midwives, existing Stage Two: Mentors as part of their mentor update and for those currently undertaking mentor training programmes to compare their experiences with the eight Stage Two: Mentors involved in the original investigation (Kinnell, 2004).

This chapter has emphasized the importance of applying research to practice and valuing the importance of qualitative data gained through interviews (Higginson, 2006; Spencer, 2007). It is envisaged that the experiences revealed by the eight mentors will help others and therefore make this chapter unique, informative and realistic. Throughout the book, a number of associated theoretical perspectives, concepts and educational frameworks have been explored in order to assist the various stages of mentors with undertaking their roles and responsibilities and as a reciprocal response, be respected as an 'effective' mentor in contemporary healthcare.

Chapter summary

This chapter has examined a number of constituent clusters and their associated elements, generated by mentors during a taped interview. Having completed this chapter you have learned about:

- what it was like becoming a mentor for the eight mentors identified in the main investigation;
- how the number of constituent clusters identified were formed as a result of a commonality between the mentors involved;
- how the mentors' qualitative statements were examined and related to some associated underpinning theoretical perspectives;
- the importance of the eight mentors sharing their experiences and how this will help other new mentors understand the reality of the role;
- how the qualitative data generated can help those undertaking mentor preparation training to understand what it means to be an effective mentor.

Mentoring nursing and healthcare students – an integrated role for all healthcare professionals

Mentorship has now become a valued role for all qualified nurses, midwives and other allied professionals. The role is now viewed as essential for establishing an effective working relationship and professional partnership between healthcare students and those with whom they work in the practice placement. Before their placement, students are introduced to the concept of mentorship and the tripartite contribution that their mentor makes towards their healthcare learning. Mentors are respected for their contribution to the effective facilitation of learning and creating an environment that is subsequently conducive to meeting the students' learning. Students are made aware, however, that the mentor has to complete their role by assessing their development, motivation and achievements of competencies, outcomes or proficiencies that are stipulated by the NMC (2004c).

Practice placement experiences hopefully give the healthcare student the opportunity to gain an insight into nursing, midwifery or any of the other allied professions. The value of mentorship relates to the theoretical concept of social learning (Bandura 1965; 1977; 1986) whereby the student can actually observe their mentor undertaking different aspects of care and the associated management of the patient and their relatives. From this direct observation the student will be able to identify their ideal role model and the professional role that they would like to emulate.

Webb and Shakespeare (2008) explored the significance of the judgements that mentors make regarding the student's ability to achieve the identified competencies, outcomes or proficiencies. They highlight the significance of 'toxic mentors', a term that was used by Darling (1985) to represent those mentors who were feeling the stress of juggling and trying to meet all the responsibilities that their role as a leader, manager and teacher incurs. There is no doubt that their role as a teacher within the mentorship process is one that mentors would like to successfully complete but at times the time constraints can be problematic, a discussion focus that is often highlighted at mentor updates.

Nevertheless, despite its challenges, mentorship is rewarding, worthwhile and brings a sense of professional achievement. Throughout this book the chapters have explored the different domains of mentorship and their associated outcomes as identified by the NMC (2008a) and also those related to the HPC (2008). There is a close resemblance in what these two main governing bodies require of their mentors in order to ensure that the healthcare student delivers safe and individualized patient care accordingly. The mentor activities, case studies and frequently asked questions have been included in order to balance an idealistic stance with reality. Mentorship requires commitment from the individual health professional but the resultant professional psychological rewards are immeasurable.

References

Ackerman, L. (1997) Development, transition or transformation: the question of change in organisations. In D. Van Eynde and J. Hoy (ed) *Organisation Development Classics*. San Francisco: Jossey Bass.

Allan, H.T., Smith, P.A. and Lorentzon, M. (2008) 'Leadership for learning: a literature study of leadership for learning in clinical practice', *Journal of Nursing Management*, 16: 545–55.

Andalo, D. (2006) 'Innovation and improvement', *Nursing Management*, 13(8): 16–17.

Anderson, E.E. and Kiger, A.M. (2008) '"I felt like a real nurse": Student nurses out on their own', *Nurse Education Today*, 28: 443–9.

Andrews, M. and Chilton, F. (2000) 'Student and mentor perceptions of mentoring effectiveness', *Nurse Education Today*, 20: 555–62.

Aston, L. (2005) 'The buddy system', *Mentors' Newsletter plus Practice Learning (PLT) News*, University of Nottingham.

Ausubel, D., Novak, J. and Hanesian, H. (1978) *Educational Psychology: A Cognitive View*. New York: Holt, Rinehart and Winston, quoted in F.M. Quinn and S.J. Hughes (2007), *Quinn's Principles and Practice of Nurse Education*, 5th edn. Cheltenham: Nelson Thornes Limited.

Bahn, D. (2001) 'Social learning theory: its application in the context of nurse education', *Nurse Education Today*, 21: 110–17.

Bandura, A. (1965) 'Influence of models' reinforcement contingencies on the acquisition of imitative responses', quoted in J.H. Donaldson and D. Carter (2005) 'The value of role modelling: perceptions of undergraduate and diploma nursing (adult) students', *Nurse Education in Practice*, 5: 353–9.

Bandura, A. (1977) 'Social learning theory', quoted in J.H. Donaldson and D. Carter (2005) 'The value of role modelling: perceptions of undergraduates and diploma nursing (adult) students', *Nurse Education in Practice*, 5: 555–62.

Bandura, A. (1986) 'Social foundations of thoughts and actions: a social cognitive theory', quoted in J.H. Donaldson and D. Carter (2005) 'The value of role modelling: perceptions of undergraduates and diploma nursing (adult) students', *Nurse Education in Practice*, 5: 555–62.

Banning, M. (2005) 'Approaches to teaching: current opinions and related research', *Nurse Education Today*, 25: 502–08.

Bloom, B. (1968) 'Learning for mastery: evaluation comment', 1(2) Center for the Study of Evaluation of Instructional Programs, Los Angeles, University of California, quoted in F.M. Quinn and S.J. Hughes (2007) *Quinn's Principles and Practice of Nurse Education*. 5th edn. Cheltenham: Nelson Thornes Limited.

Bondy, K.N. (1983) 'Criterion-referenced definitions for rating scales in clinical education', *Criteria in Clinical Evaluation*, 22(9): 376–82.

Borlase, J. and Abelson-Mitchell, N. (2008) 'User perception of the knowledge underpinning practice orientation dial (KUPOD) as a tool to enhance learning', *Nurse Education in Practice*, 8: 9–19.

Bradshaw, A. (1998) 'Defining "competency" in nursing (part two) an analytical review', *Journal of Clinical Nursing*, 7: 103–11.

Bradshaw, B. (2008) *NHS Choices: Delivering for the NHS*. London: NHS Choices.

Bray, L. and Nettleton, P. (2007) 'Assessor or mentor? Role confusion in professional education', *Nurse Education Today*, 27: 848–55.

Brennan, A.M. and Hutt, R. (2001) 'The challenges and conflicts of facilitating learning in practice: the experience of two clinical educators', *Nurse Education in Practice*, 1: 181–8.

British Dyslexia Association (2007) *What is Dyslexia?* Accessed 28.10.08 www.bdadyslexia.org.uk/whatisdyslexiap.html

Brown, S.J. (2008) *Evidence-Based Nursing: The Research-Practice Connection*. London: Jones and Bartlett Publishers.

Burnard, P. (2005) 'Interviewing', *Nurse Researcher*, 13(1): 4–6.

Burns, N. and Grove, S.K. (2007) *Understanding Nursing Research: Building an Evidence-based Practice*, 4th edn. Philadelphia, PA: Saunders.

Calman, L., Watson, R., Norman, I., Redfern, S. and Murrells, T. (2002) 'Assessing practice of student nurses: methods, preparation of assessors and student views', *Journal of Advanced Nursing*, 38(5): 516–23.

Carr, G. (2008) 'Changes in nurse education: delivering the curriculum', *Nurse Education Today*, 28: 120–7.

Castledine, G. (2008) 'Are we witnessing the deterioration of nursing?' *British Journal of Nursing*, 17(15).

Chan, D. (2001) 'Development of an innovative tool to assess hospital learning environments', *Nurse Education Today*, 21: 624–31.

Clark, L. (2008) 'Clinical leadership: values, beliefs and vision', *Nursing Management*, 15(7): 30–5.

Clarke, A. (2006) 'Qualitative interview: encountering ethical issues and challenges', *Nurse Researcher*, 13(4): 19–29.

Clarke, K. and Iphofen, R. (2006) 'Issues in phenomenological nursing research: the combined use of pain diaries and interviewing', *Nurse Researcher*, 13(3): 62–74.

Clore, G.L. (1994) in R. Gross (2001) 'Emotion: understanding the role of cognitive factors', *Psychology Review*, November: 10–13.

Clynes, M.P. and Raftery, S.E.C. (2008) 'Feedback: an essential element of student learning in clinical practice', *Nurse Education in Practice*, 8: 405–11.

Cohen, L. and Manion, L. (2007) *Research Methods in Education*, 6th edn. London: Routledge.

Cole, M. (2006) 'Using motivational paradigm to improve hand washing compliance', *Nurse Education in Practice*, 6: 156–62.

Corben, V. (1999) 'Misusing phenomenology in nursing research: identifying the issues', *Nurse Researcher*, 6(3): 52–66.

Corlett, J. (2000) 'The perceptions of nurse teachers, student nurses and preceptors of the theory–practice gap in nurse education', *Nurse Education Today*, 20: 499–505.

Cormack, D. (ed.) (2000) *The Research Process in Nursing*, 4th edn. Oxford: Blackwell Sciences.

Darling, L.A. (1985) 'What to do about toxic mentors', *Journal of Nursing Administration*, 5: 43–44.

Davies, I.K. (1981) *Instructional Technique*. New York: McGraw-Hill Book Company.

Department of Health (DH) (1989) *Working for Patients*. London: HMSO.

Department of Health (DH) (1991) *Research for Health: A Research and Development Strategy for the NHS.* London: HMSO.

Department of Health (DH) (1996a) *Promoting Clinical Effectiveness: A Framework for Action In and Through the NHS.* Leeds: Department of Health.

Department of Health (DH) (1996b) *Research and Development: Towards an Evidence Based Health Service.* London: HMSO.

Department of Health (DH) (1997) *The New NHS: Modern and Dependable.* London: HMSO.

Department of Health (DH) (1998) *A First Class Service: Quality in the New NHS.* London: HMSO.

Department of Health (DH) (1999) *Making a Difference: Strengthening the Nursing, Midwifery and Health Visiting Contribution to Health and Healthcare.* London: Department of Health.

Department of Health (DH) (2000) *The NHS Plan: A Plan for Investment, A Plan for Reform.* London: Department of Health.

Department of Health (DH) (2004) *The NHS Knowledge and Skills Framework (NHS KSF) and the Development Review Process.* London: Department of Health.

Department of Health (DH) (2008) *NHS Next Stage Review.* London: Department of Health.

Department of Health (DH) (2009a) *Tackling Concerns Nationally: Establishing the Office of the Health Professions Adjudicator.* London: Department of Health.

Department of Health (DH) (2009b) *Tackling Concerns Locally: Report of the Working Group.* London: Department of Health.

Dolan, G. (2003) 'Assessing student nurse clinical competency: will we ever get it right?' *Journal of Clinical Nursing,* 12: 132–41.

Donaldson, J.H. and Carter, D. (2005) 'The value of role modelling: perceptions of undergraduate and diploma nursing (adult) students', *Nurse Education in Practice,* 5: 353–9.

Downie, C. and Basford, P. (eds) (2003) *Teaching and Assessing in Clinical Practice: A Reader.* Reprinted. London: Greenwich University Press.

Duffy, K. (2004) *Failing Students: A Qualitative Study of Factors that Influence the Decisions Regarding Assessment of Students' Competence in Practice.* Glasgow: Caledonian University.

Duffy, K. and Hardicre, J. (2007a) 'Supporting failing students in practice – 1: Assessment', *Nursing Times,* 103(47): 28–9.

Duffy, K. and Hardicre, J. (2007b) 'Supporting failing students in practice – 2: Management', *Nursing Times,* 103(48): 28–9.

Edwards, C. (2001) 'New education and training supports clinical effectiveness in nursing and allied health professionals', *Clinical Effectiveness in Nursing,* 5: 1–3.

Egan, G. (2007) *The Skilled Helper,* 8th edn. Monterey, CA: Brooks/Cole.

Eisner, D. (1975) *Instructional and Expressive Objectives in Curriculum Design.* London: Croom Helm.

Elcock, K. and Sookhoo, D. (2007) 'Evaluating a new role to support mentors in practice', www.nursingtimes.net

English National Board for Nursing and Midwifery/Department of Health (2001) *Placements in Focus: Guidance for Education in Practice for Health Care Professionals.* London: E.N.B./D.H.

Eysenck, M. (2002) *Simply Psychology,* 2nd edn. Hove: Psychology Press Limited.

Foundation of Nursing Studies (2001) *Taking Action: Moving Towards Evidence Based Practice – Main Report*. London: Foundation of Nursing Studies.

Fowler, J., Jarvis, P. and Chevannes, M. (2002) *Practical Statistics for Nursing and Health Care*. Chichester: Wiley.

Fretwell, J.E. (1982) Ward teaching and learning: Sister and the learning environment. London, RCN, quoted in H.T. Allan, P.A. Smith and M. Lorentzon (2008) 'Leadership for learning: a literature study of leadership for learning in clinical practice', *Journal of Nursing Management*, 16: 545–55.

Freud, S. (1923) *The Ego and the Id*. Harmondsworth: Pelican, cited in R. Gross (2005) *Psychology: The Science of Mind and Behaviour*, 5th edn. London: Hodder Arnold.

Fulton, J., Bohler, A., Storm Hansen, G., Kauffeldt, A., Welander, E., Reis Santos, M., Thorarinsdottir, K. and Ziarko, E. (2008) 'Mentorship: an international perspective', *Nurse Education in Practice*, 7: 399–406.

Gerrish, K. and Lacey, A. (eds) (2006) *The Research Process in Nursing*, 5th edn. Oxford: Blackwell Publishers.

Gerrish, K. and McMahon, A. (2006) 'Research and development in nursing', in K. Gerrish and A. Lacey (eds) *The Research Process in Nursing*, 5th edn. Oxford: Blackwell Publishers.

Greenhalgh, T. (1997) 'How to read a paper: assessing the methodological quality of published papers', *British Medical Journal*, 315: 305–08.

Greenhalgh, T. (2006) *How to Read a Paper: The Basics of Evidence-based Medicine*, 3rd edn. Oxford/Malden, MA: BMJ Books.

Gross, R. (2005) *Psychology: The Science of Mind and Behaviour*, 5th edn. London: Hodder Arnold.

Hallett, C. (1995) 'Understanding the phenomenological approach to research', *Nurse Researcher*, 3(2): 55–65.

Harris, H. and Inayat, Q. (1997) 'Semi-structured interview schedules for gathering psychosocial health data', *Nurse Researcher*, 5(1): 73–85.

Hartley, J. and Allison, M. (2002) 'The role of leadership in the modernisation and improvement of public services', in Taylor, V. (2007) 'Leadership for service improvement', *Nursing Management*, 13(9): 30–4.

Hayes, N. (2005) *Foundations of Psychology*, 3rd edn. Reprinted. London: Thomson.

Health and Safety Executive (1974) *Health and Safety Law*. Suffolk: Health and Safety Executive.

Health Professions Council (2004) *Standards of Proficiency: Operating Department Practitioners*. London: HPC.

Health Professions Council (2005) *A Disabled Person's Guide to Becoming a Health Professional: Consultative Document*. London: HPC.

Health Professions Council (2007a) *A Guide for Employers and Registrants: Managing Fitness to Practice*. London: HPC.

Health Professions Council (2007b) *Your Duties as a Registrant: Standards of Conduct, Performance and Ethics*. London: HPC.

Health Professions Council (2007c) *Standards of Proficiency: Dietitians*. London: HPC.

Health Professions Council (2007d) *Standards of Proficiency: Occupational Therapists*. London: HPC.

Health Professions Council (2007e) *Standards of Proficiency: Physiotherapists*. London: HPC.

Health Professions Council (2007f) *Standards of Proficiency: Speech and Language Therapists*. London: HPC.

Health Professions Council (2007g) *A Guide for Prospective Registrants and Admissions Staff: A Disabled Person's Guide to Becoming a Health Professional*. London: HPC.

Health Professions Council (2008) *Your Duties as a Registrant: Standards of Conduct, Performance and Ethics*. London: HPC.

Higginson, R. (2004) 'The theory-practice gap still exists in nursing education', *British Journal of Nursing*, 13(20): 1168.

Higginson, R. (2006) 'Fears, worries and experiences of first year pre-registration students: a qualitative study', *Nurse Researcher*, 13(3): 32–49.

Hinchliff, S. (2009) *The Practitioner as Teacher*, 4th edn. Edinburgh: Churchill Livingstone.

Holloway, I. and Fulbrook, P. (2001) 'Revisiting qualitative inquiry: interviewing in nursing and midwifery research', *Research*, 6(1): 539–50.

Honey, P. and Mumford, A. (1989) 'Setting the scene for learning styles', in P. Honey and A. Mumford, *Manual of Learning Styles*. Berkshire: Honey.

Hurley, C. and Snowden, S. (2008) 'Mentoring in times of change', *British Association of Critical Care Nurses*, 269–75.

Hutchings, A., Williamson, G. and Humphreys, A. (2005) 'Supporting learners in clinical practice: capacity issues', *Journal of Clinical Nursing*, 14(8): 945–-55.

Iles, V. and Sutherland, K. (2001) *Managing Change in the NHS: Organisational Change, A Review for Health Care Managers, Professionals and Researchers*. London: National Co-ordinating Centre for NHS Service Delivery and Organisation.

Jones, A. (2008a) 'Friends in higher places: we need to know more about the benefits or otherwise from peer mentoring in nursing curricula', *Nurse Education Today*, 28: 261–3.

Jones, L. (2008b) 'Leadership in the "new" NHS', *Nursing Management*, 15(6): 32–5.

Jordan, K., Ong, B.N. and Croft, P. (1998) *Mastering Statistics*. Cheltenham: Stanley Thornes.

Jowett, S. and McMullan, M. (2007) 'Learning in practice – practice educator role', *Nurse Education in Practice*. 7: 266–71.

Kenmore, P. (2008) 'Exploring leadership styles', *Nursing Management*, 15(1): 24–6.

Kerridge, J.L. (2008) 'Supporting student nurses on placement in nursing homes: the challenges for the link-tutor role', *Nurse Education in Practice*, 8: 389–96.

Kinnell, D. (2004) 'An interpretive phenomenological investigation into the experience, of qualified nurses acting as a mentor in contemporary health care settings', unpublished MSc dissertation, Manchester University.

Kitson, A.C. (2001) 'Does nursing education have a future?', *Nurse Education Today*, 212: 86–96.

Knowles, M. (1984) 'Introduction: the art and science of helping adults learn', in C. Downie and P. Basford (eds) (2003) *Teaching and Assessing in Clinical Practice: A Reader*, 2nd edn, Reprinted. London: University of Greenwich Press.

Knowles, M. (1994) *The Adult Learner: A Neglected Species*, 4th edn, Reprinted. Houston, TX: Gulf Publishing.

Koch, T. (1995) 'Interpretive approaches in nursing research: the influence of Husserl and Heidegger', *Journal of Advanced Nursing*, 21(5): 827–36.

Koch, T. (1999) 'Phenomenology revisited: an interpretive research process: revisiting phenomenological and hermeneutical approaches', *Nurse Researcher*, 6(3): 20–34.

Koh, L.C. (2002) 'The perceptions of nursing students of practice-based teaching', *Nurse Education in Practice*, 2: 35–43.

Kolb, D.A. (1976) 'The Learning Style Inventory: Technical Manual', in F.M. Quinn and S.J. Hughes (2007) *Quinn's Principles and Practice of Nurse Education*. Cheltenham: Nelson Thornes Limited.

Kopp, P. (2001) 'Fit for practice – part 3.3: health care interactions', *Nursing Times*, 97(12): 47–50.

Landers, M.G. (2000) 'The theory-practice gap in nursing: the role of the nurse teacher', *Journal of Advanced Nursing*, 32(6): 1550–6.

Levett-Jones, T. and Lathlean, J. (2008) 'Belongingness: a prerequisite for nursing students' clinical learning', *Nurse Education in Practice*, 8: 103–11.

Levinson, D.J., Darrow, D.N., Klein, E.B., Levinson, M.H. and McKee, B. (1978) *The Seasons of a Man's Life*. New York: A.A. Knopf, quoted in R. Gross (2005) *Psychology: The Science of Mind and Behaviour*, 5th edn. London: Hodder Arnold.

Lewin, K. (1951) Field Theory in Social Science. New York, Harper Row, quoted in Iles, V., Sutherland, K. (2001) *Managing Change in the NHS. Organizational Change, A Review for Health Care Managers, Professional and Researchers*. London: National coordinating centre for NHS Service Delivery and Organisation.

Lindsay, G.M. (2006) 'Experiencing nursing education research: narrative inquiry and interpretive phenomenology', *Nurse Researcher*, 13(4): 30–47.

Lloyd Jones, M., Walters, S. and Akehurst, R. (2001) 'The implications of contact with the mentor for pre-registration nursing and midwifery students', *Journal of Advanced Nursing*, 35(2): 151–60.

Maher, L. (2006) in Andalo, D. (2006) 'Innovation and improvement', *Nursing Management*, 13(8): 16–17.

Marquis, B.L. and Huston, C.J. (2006) *Leadership Roles and Management Functions in Nursing*, 5th edn. Philadelphia, PA: Lippincott, Williams and Wilkins.

Martin, G.W. and Mitchell, G. (2001) 'A study of critical incident analysis as a route to the identification of change necessary in clinical practice: addressing the theory–practice gap', *Nurse Education in Practice*, 1(1): 27–34.

Maslow, A. (1954) *Motivation and Personality*. New York: Harper and Row.

Maslow, A. (1970) *Motivation and Personality*, 2nd edn. New York: Harper and Row

Mason, T. and Whitehead, E. (2004) *Thinking Nursing*. Maidenhead: Open University Press.

Mathews, N. and Chu Huang, Y. (2004) quoted in P.A. Crookes and S. Davies (eds) (2004) *Research in Practice: Essential Skills for Reading and Applying Research in Nursing Care*. London: Bailliere Tindall.

McCann, T. and Clark, E. (2005) 'Using unstructured interviews with participants who have schizophrenia', *Nurse Researcher*, 13(1): 7–18.

McEwan, M. (2006a) 'Philosophy, science and nursing', quoted in M. McEwan and E.M. Wills (eds) *Theoretical Basis for Nursing*, Philadelphia, PA: Lippincott, Williams and Wilkins.

McEwan, M. (2006b) 'Application of theory in nursing practice', quoted in M. McEwan and E.M. Wills (eds) *Theoretical Basis for Nursing*, Philadelphia, PA: Lippincott, Williams and Wilkins.

McEwan, M. and Wills, E.M. (2006) *Theoretical Basis for Nursing.* Philadelphia, PA: Lippincott, Williams and Wilkins.

Menix, K.D. (2003) 'Leading change', quoted in P.S. Yoder-Wise, (ed) *Leading and Managing in Nursing*, 3rd edn. St Louis: Mosby.

Midgley, K. (2006) 'Pre-registration student nurses' perception of the hospital-learning environment during clinical placements', *Nurse Education Today*, 26: 338–45.

Moore, D. (2005) *Assuring Fitness for Practice: A Policy Review Commissioned by the Nursing and Midwifery Council Nursing Task and Finish Group.* London: NMC.

Moores, B. and Moulton, A. (1979) Patterns of nurse activity. *Journal of Advanced Nursing.* 4(2): 137–49, quoted in H.T. Allan, P.A. Smith and M. Lorentzon (2008) 'Leadership for learning: a literature study of leadership for learning in clinical practice'. *Journal of Nursing Management*, 16: 545–55.

Morton-Cooper, A. and Palmer, A. (2000) *Mentoring, Preceptorship and Clinical Supervision: A Guide to Professional Roles in Clinical Practice*, 2nd edn. London: Blackwell Science.

Moseley, L.G. and Davies, M. (2007) 'What do mentors find difficult?' *Journal of Clinical Nursing*, 17(12): 1627–34.

Murphy-Black, T. (2000) 'Questionnaire', quoted in D. Cormack (ed.) *The Research Process in Nursing*, 4th edn. Oxford: Blackwell Sciences.

Murray, C., Grant, M.J., Howarth, M.L. and Leigh, J. (2008) 'The use of simulation as a teaching and learning approach to support practice learning', *Nurse Education in Practice*, 8: 5–8.

Myall, M., Levett-Jones, T. and Lathlean, J. (2008) 'Mentorship in contemporary practice: the experience of nursing students and practice mentors', *Journal of Clinical Nursing*, 17: 1834–42.

Neary, M. (2001) 'Responsive assessment: assessing student nurses' clinical competence', *Nurse Education Today*, 21: 3–17.

Nettleton, P. and Bray, L. (2008) 'Current mentorship schemes might be doing our students a disservice', *Nurse Education in Practice*, 8: 205–12.

Newell, R. and Burnard, P. (2006) *Vital Notes for Nurses: Research for Evidence-Based Practice.* Oxford: Blackwell Publishing Limited.

NHS Choices (2008) *NHS Choices: Delivering for the NHS.* London: NHS Choices.

NHS Connecting for Health (2009) *Learning to Manage Health Information: A Theme for Clinical Education: Making a Difference.* London: NHS Connecting for Health.

NHS Institute for Innovation and Improvement (2006) *NHS Leadership Qualities Framework.* www.NHSLeadershipQualities.nhs.uk

NHS Institute for Innovation and Improvement (2007) *Improvement Leaders' Guide: Matching Capacity and Demand – Process and Systems Thinking.* Coventry: NHS Institute for Innovation and Improvement.

Nicklin, P.J. and Kenworthy, N. (2000) *Teaching and Assessing in Nursing Practice: An Experimental Approach*, 3rd edn. London: Bailliere Tindall.

Nursing and Midwifery Council (NMC) (2004a) *Standards for the Preparation of Teachers of Nurses, Midwives and Specialist Public Health Nurses.* London: NMC.

Nursing and Midwifery Council (NMC) (2004b) *The NMC Code of Professional Conduct: Standards for Conduct, Performance and Ethics.* London: NMC.

Nursing and Midwifery Council (NMC) (2004c) *Standards of Proficiency for Pre-Registration Nursing Education.* London: NMC.

Nursing and Midwifery Council (NMC) (2006a) *Standards to Support Learning and Assessment in Practice: NMC Standards for Mentors, Practice Teachers and Teachers.* London: NMC.

Nursing and Midwifery Council (NMC) (2006b) *Standards for the Preparation and Practice of Supervisors of Midwives.* London: NMC.

Nursing and Midwifery Council (NMC) (2007a) *Guidance for the Introduction of the Essential Skills Clusters for Pre-registration Nursing Programmes: Annexe to NMC Circular 07/2007.* www.nmc-uk.org

Nursing and Midwifery Council (NMC) (2007b) *Essential Skills Clusters (ESCs) for Pre-registration Nursing Programmes: Annexe 2 to NMC Circular 07/2007.* www.nmc-uk.org

Nursing and Midwifery Council (NMC) (2007c) *Mapping of Essential Skills Clusters to the Standards of Proficiency for Pre-Registration Nursing Education (NMC 2004): Annexe 3 to NMC Circular 07/2007.* www.nmc-uk.org

Nursing and Midwifery Council (NMC) (2008a) *Standards to Support Learning and Assessment in Practice: NMC Standards for Mentors, Practice Teachers and Teachers,* 2nd edn. London: NMC.

Nursing and Midwifery Council (NMC) (2008b) *The Code: Standards of Conduct, Performance and Ethics for Nurses and Midwives.* London: NMC.

Nursing and Midwifery Council (NMC) (2008c) *A Review of Pre-registration Nursing Education: Report of Consultation Findings.* London: NMC.

Nursing and Midwifery Council (NMC) (2008d) *Standards for Medicines Management.* London: NMC.

Nursing and Midwifery Council (NMC) (2008e) *The Prep Handbook.* London: NMC.

Nursing and Midwifeery Council (NMC) (2009) *Guidance on Professional Conduct for Nursing and Midwifery Student.* London: NMC.

Oliver, R., Endersby, C. (2003) *Teaching and Assessing Nurses: A Handbook for Preceptors.* London: Bailliere Tindall.

Parkinson, B. (1997) 'Emotion', quoted in B. Parkinson and A.M. Colman (eds) *Emotion and Motivation.* London: Longman Essential Psychology.

Parliament (1995) Disability Discrimination Act. London: HMSO.

Parliament (2001) Special Educational Needs and Disability Act. London: HMSO.

Parliament (2005) Disability Discrimination Act. London: HMSO.

Pavlov, I. (1927) *Conditional Reflexes.* Oxford: Oxford University Press, quoted in R. Gross (2005) *Psychology: The Science of Mind and Behaviour,* 5th edn. London: Hodder Arnold.

Pearce, C. (2007) 'Ten steps to staff motivation', *Nursing Management,* 13(9): 21.

Pettinger, R. (2007) *Introduction to Management,* 4th edn. Basingstoke: Palgrave.

Piaget, J. (1963) *The Origins of Intelligence in Children.* New York: Norton, quoted in R. Gross (2005) *Psychology: The Science of Mind and Behaviour,* 5th edn. London: Hodder Arnold.

Polit, D.F. and Beck, C.T. (2006) *Essentials of Nursing Research: Methods, Appraisal, and Utilization,* 6th edn. London: Lippincott, Williams and Wilkins.

Polit, D.F. and Hungler, B.P. (1999) *Essentials of Nursing Research: Methods, Appraisal and Utilization,* 4th edn. Philadelphia, PA: Lippincott.

Porter, S. and Carter, D.F. (2000) 'Common terms and concepts in research', cited in D. Cormack (2000) *The Research Process in Nursing,* 4th edn. Oxford: Blackwell Sciences.

Pulsford, D., Boit, K. and Owens, S. (2002) 'Are mentors ready to make a difference?: a survey of mentors' attitudes towards nurse education' *Nurse Education Today*, 22: 439–46.

Quinn, F.M. and Hughes, S.J. (2007) *Quinn's Principles and Practice of Nurse Education*, 5th edn. Cheltenham: Nelson Thornes Limited.

Rogers, C. (1951) quoted in P. Morrison and P. Burnard (1993) *Caring and Communicating: The Interpersonal Relationship in Nursing*. Reprinted. London: Macmillan.

Rogers, C. (1969) *Freedom to Learn*. Columbus, OH: Merrill, quoted in F.M. Quinn and S.J. Hughes (2007) *Quinn's Principles and Practice of Nurse Education*, 5th edn. Cheltenham: Nelson Thornes Limited.

Rogers, C. (1983) *Freedom to Learn in the '80's*. Columbus, OH: Charles Merrill, quoted in R. Gross (2005) *Psychology: The Science of Mind and Behaviour*, 5th edn. London: Hodder Arnold.

Rosenberg, M.J. and Hovland, C.I. (1960) 'Cognitive, affective and behavioural components of attitude', quoted in R. Gross (2005) *Psychology: The Science of Mind and Behaviour*, 5th edn. London: Hodder Arnold.

Rowntree, D. (1997) *Assessing Students: How Shall We Know Them?* Reprinted. London: Harper Row.

Royal College of Nursing (RCN) (2004) *Helping Students Get the Best from their Practice Placements: A Royal College of Nursing Toolkit*. Reprinted. London: RCN.

Royal College of Nursing (RCN) (2007a) *Information for Student Nurses: Outlining the NHS Knowledge and Skills Framework*. London: RCN.

Royal College of Nursing (RCN) (2007b) *Guidance for Mentors of Nursing Students and Midwives: An RCN Toolkit*, 2nd edn. London: RCN.

Sines, D., Harris, D., Firth, J., Boden, L. (2006) 'Ensuring fitness for practice', *Nursing Management*, 13(8): 28–31.

Skills for Health (2008) *EQuIP: Enhancing Quality in Partnership, Healthcare Education QA Framework*. Leeds: Skills for Health.

Skinner, B. (1938) *The Behaviour of Organisms*. New York: Appleton-Century-Crofts, quoted in R. Gross (2005) *Psychology: The Science of Mind and Behaviour*, 5th edn. London: Hodder Arnold.

Spencer, L.H. (2007) 'Using cluster analysis to explore survey data', *Nurse Researcher*, 15(1): 37–54.

Spouse, J. (2001) 'Work-based learning in health care environments', *Nurse Education in Practice*, 1: 12–18.

Stommel, M. and Wills, C.E. (2004) *Clinical Research: Principles for Advanced Practice Nurses*. London: Lippincott, Williams and Wilkins.

Taylor, B. (1995) 'Interpreting phenomenology for nursing research', *Nurse Researcher*, 3(2): 66–79.

Taylor, V. (2007) 'Leadership for service improvement', *Nursing Management*, 13(9): 30–4.

Thorsteinsson, L.S. (2002) 'The quality of nursing care as perceived by individuals with chronic illnesses: the magical touch of nursing', *Journal of Clinical Nursing*, 11: 32–40.

Timmins, F. (2008) *Making Sense of Portfolios: A Guide for Nursing Students*. Maidenhead: Open University Press.

Tomey, A.M. (2004) *Guide to Nursing Management and Leadership*. 7th edn. St Louis: Mosby.

Topping, A. (2006) 'The quantitative-qualitative continuum', in K. Gerrish and A. Lacey (eds) *The Research Process in Nursing*. Oxford: Blackwell Publishing.

Turkington, C. and Harris, J.R. (2006) *The A to Z of Learning Disabilities*. New York: Checkmark Books.

United Kingdom Central Council for Nursing, Midwifery and Health Visiting (1999) *Fitness for Practice: The UKCC Commission for Nursing and Midwifery Education*. London: U.K.C.C.

University of Nottingham (2006) *University Disability Equality Scheme for the University of Nottingham, 2006–2009*. Nottingham: The University of Nottingham.

van der Gaag, A. (2008) *Your Duties as a Registrant: Standards of Conduct, Performance and Ethics*. London: Health Professions Council.

Walker, W. (2007) 'Ethical consideration in phenomenological research', *Nurse Researcher*, 14(3): 36–45.

Watson, N.A. (1999) 'Mentoring today – the student's views: an investigative case study of pre-registration nursing students' experiences and perceptions of mentoring in one theory/practice module of the Common Foundation Programme on a Project 2000 course', *Journal of Advanced Nursing*, 29(1): 254–62.

Watson, H.E. and Harris, B. (2000) *Supporting Students in Practice Placements in Scotland*. Glasgow: Glasgow Caledonian University and National Board for Nursing, Midwifery and Health Visiting for Scotland.

Watson, S. (2000) 'The support that mentors receive in the clinical setting', *Nurse Education Today*, 20: 585–92.

Watson, S. (2004) 'Mentor preparation: reasons for undertaking the course and *expectations* of the candidates', *Nurse Education Today*, 24: 30–40.

Webb, C. and Shakespeare, P. (2008) 'Judgements about mentoring relationships in nursing', *Nurse Education Today*, 28(5): 563–71.

Welch, R.A. (1999) 'Problem solving and decision making', quoted in P.S. Yoder-Wise (ed), *Leading and Managing in Nursing*, 2nd edn. London: Mosby.

Whyte, L. (2007) 'Applied leadership: the team wheel', *Nursing Management*, 13(9): 22–4.

Wiener, B. (1979) 'A theory of motivation for some classroom experiences', *Journal of Educational Psychology*, 71: 3–25.

Wilkinson, J. (1999) 'A practical guide to assessing nursing students in clinical practice', *British Journal of Nursing*, 8(4): 218–22.

Wilson-Barnett, J., Butterworth, T., White, E., Twinn, S., Davies, S. and Riley, L. (1995) 'Clinical support and the Project 2000 student: factors influencing this process', *Journal of Advanced Nursing*, 21: 1152–8.

Index

This index is in word-by-word order. Page references in *italics* indicate boxes, those in **bold** indicate tables, and those in ***bold italics*** indicate figures.